Minimally Invasive Hand Surgery

Editor

CATHERINE CURTIN

HAND CLINICS

www.hand.theclinics.com

Consulting Editor
KEVIN C. CHUNG

February 2014 • Volume 30 • Number 1

ELSEVIER

1600 John F. Kennedy Boulevard • Suite 1800 • Philadelphia, Pennsylvania, 19103-2899

http://www.theclinics.com

HAND CLINICS Volume 30, Number 1
February 2014 ISSN 0749-0712, ISBN-13: 978-0-323-26658-1

Editor: Jennifer Flynn-Briggs
Developmental editor: Stephanie Carter

Hand Clinics (ISSN 0749-0712) is published quarterly by Elsevier Inc., 360 Park Avenue South, New York, NY 10010-1710. Months of publication are February, May, August, and November. Business and Editorial Offices: 1600 John F. Kennedy Blvd., Ste. 1800, Philadelphia, PA 19103-2899. Customer Service Office: 3251 Riverport Lane, Maryland Heights, MO 63043. Periodicals postage paid at New York, NY and at additional mailing offices. Subscription price is $390.00 per year (domestic individuals), $606.00 per year (domestic institutions), $194.00 per year (domestic students/residents), $445.00 per year (Canadian individuals), $691.00 per year (Canadian institutions), $530.00 per year (international individuals), $691.00 per year (international institutions), and $256.00 per year (international and Canadian students/residents). Foreign air speed delivery is included in all *Clinics* subscription prices. All prices are subject to change without notice. **POSTMASTER:** Send address changes to *Hand Clinics*, Elsevier Health Sciences Division, Subscription Customer Service, 3251 Riverport Lane, Maryland Heights, MO 63043. Customer Service (orders, claims, online, change of address): Elsevier Health Sciences Division, Subscription Customer Service, 3251 Riverport Lane, Maryland Heights, MO 63043. Tel: 1-800-654-2452 (U.S. and Canada); 314-447-8871 (outside U.S. and Canada). Fax: 314-447-8029. E-mail: journalscustomerservice-usa@elsevier.com (for print support); journalsonlinesupport-usa@elsevier.com (for online support).

Reprints. For copies of 100 or more of articles in this publication, please contact the Commercial Reprints Department, Elsevier Inc., 360 Park Avenue South, New York, New York 10010-1710. Tel.: 212-633-3874; Fax: 212-633-3820; E-mail: reprints@elsevier.com.

Hand Clinics is covered in *MEDLINE/PubMed (Index Medicus), Current Contents/Clinical Medicine, EMBASE/Excerpta Medica,* and *ISI/BIOMED.*

Printed and bound by CPI Group (UK) Ltd, Croydon, CR0 4YY

Transferred to digital print 2012

Contributors

CONSULTING EDITOR

KEVIN C. CHUNG, MD, MS
Charles B.G. de Nancrede Professor of Surgery, Section of Plastic Surgery, Department of Surgery, Assistant Dean for Faculty Affairs, Associate Director of Global REACH, University of Michigan Medical School, University of Michigan Health System, Ann Arbor, Michigan

EDITOR

CATHERINE CURTIN, MD
Assistant Professor of Plastic Surgery, Surgery Department, Palo Alto Veterans Hospital, Palo Alto, California

AUTHORS

JOSHUA M. ADKINSON, MD
Division of Plastic Surgery, Department of Surgery, Lehigh Valley Health Network, Allentown, Pennsylvania

WALTER MANNA ALBERTONI, PhD, Habilitation (professorship) in Orthopedics
Associate Professor, Discipline of Hand and Upper Limb Surgery, Department of Orthopedics and Traumatology, UNIFESP – Federal University of São Paulo, São Paulo City, São Paulo, Brazil

KELLI NICOLE BELANGEE WEBB, MD
PGY 6 Plastic Surgery Resident, SIU School of Medicine, Springfield, Illinois

JOÃO CARLOS BELLOTI, PhD, Doctoral degree in Orthopedics
Associate Professor, Discipline of Hand and Upper Limb Surgery, Department of Orthopedics and Traumatology, UNIFESP – Federal University of São Paulo, São Paulo City, São Paulo, Brazil

NICHOLAS A. BONTEMPO, MD
Warren Alpert Medical School of Brown University, Providence, Rhode Island

KEVIN C. CHUNG, MD, MS
Charles B.G. de Nancrede Professor of Surgery, Section of Plastic Surgery, Department of Surgery, Assistant Dean for Faculty Affairs, Associate Director of Global REACH, University of Michigan Medical School, University of Michigan Health System, Ann Arbor, Michigan

CATHERINE CURTIN, MD
Assistant Professor of Plastic Surgery, Surgery Department, Palo Alto Veterans Hospital, Palo Alto, California

ROBERTO DIAZ, MD
Orthopaedics Department, Stanford University, Palo Alto, California

FLAVIO FALOPPA, PhD, Habilitation (professorship) in Orthopedics
Associate Professor, Discipline of Hand and Upper Limb Surgery, Department of Orthopedics and Traumatology, UNIFESP – Federal University of São Paulo, São Paulo City, São Paulo, Brazil

LESLIE TZE FUNG LEUNG, BSc(Pharm), MD
Plastic Surgery Resident, University of British Columbia, Vancouver, British of Colombia, Canada

JOÃO BAPTISTA GOMES DOS SANTOS, PhD, Doctoral degree in Orthopedics
Associate Professor, Head of Upper Limb and Hand Surgery Team, Discipline of Hand and Upper Limb Surgery, Department of Orthopedics and Traumatology, UNIFESP – Federal University of São Paulo, São Paulo City, São Paulo, Brazil

SOL GREGORY, BHK, MD
Plastic Surgery Resident, University of British Columbia, Vancouver, British of Colombia, Canada

TORBEN B. HANSEN, MD, PhD
Section of Hand Surgery, Department of Orthopaedics, Regional Hospital Holstebro, Holstebro, Denmark; Aarhus University, Aarhus C, Denmark

VINCENT R. HENTZ, MD
Professor of Surgery (Emeritus), Robert A. Chase Center for Hand and Upper Limb Surgery, Stanford University, Palo Alto, California

DON LALONDE, MD, MSc, FRCSC
Professor, Surgery, Dalhousie University, Saint John, New Brunswick, Canada

DONALD H. LALONDE, MD, MSc, FRCSC
Professor, Surgery, Dalhousie University, Hilyard Place, Saint John, Canada

HAIDER GHALIB MAJEED, MD
Section of Hand Surgery, Department of Orthopaedics, Regional Hospital Holstebro, Holstebro, Denmark

ARASH MOMENI, MD
Division of Plastic and Reconstructive Surgery, Stanford University Medical Center, Stanford, California

MICHAEL W. NEUMEISTER, MD, FRCSC, FACS
Professor & Chair, SIU School of Medicine, Springfield, Illinois

JOSEPH M. PIROLO, MD
Department of Orthopaedic Surgery, Stanford University Medical Center, Stanford

MICHAEL ROMANELLI, BS
SIU School of Medicine, Springfield, Illinois

EDSON SASAHARA SATO, PhD, Doctoral degree in Orthopedics
Team Surgeon, Discipline of Hand and Upper Limb Surgery, Department of Orthopedics and Traumatology, UNIFESP – Federal University of São Paulo, São Paulo City, São Paulo, Brazil

DAVID J. SLUTSKY, MD
Associate Professor, Department of Orthopedics, Harbor-UCLA Medical Center, The Hand and Wrist Institute, Torrance, California

JULIEN TREVARE
Culver city, California

ARNOLD-PETER C. WEISS, MD
Warren Alpert Medical School of Brown University, Providence, Rhode Island

JEFFREY YAO, MD
Associate Professor, Department of Orthopaedic Surgery, Robert A. Chase Hand and Upper Limb Center, Stanford University Medical Center, Stanford

HORST ZAJONC, MD
Department of Plastic and Hand Surgery, University of Freiburg Medical Center, Freiburg, Germany

Contents

Preface ix

Catherine Curtin

Minimally Invasive Anesthesia in Wide Awake Hand Surgery 1

Don Lalonde

Videos of how to inject carpal tunnel with minimal pain for wide awake surgery; Field sterility for surgery; surgery; intraoperative patient advice; bandage; and typical patient impression after surgery accompany this article

The minimally invasive tumescent local anesthesia technique used in wide-awake hand surgery is having an impact in hand surgery practice. Patients spend less time and money and get to speak to their surgeon and receive education during the surgery itself. Improvements in operations such as flexor tendon repair have happened, because surgeons can see movement during the case and make adjustments before the skin is closed. Surgeons can perform more cases in the same amount of time with fewer personnel. The cost of the surgery is decreased, as all expenses surrounding the provision of sedation are removed.

Minimally Invasive Finger Fracture Management: Wide-awake Closed Reduction, K-wire Fixation, and Early Protected Movement 7

Sol Gregory, Donald H. Lalonde, and Leslie Tze Fung Leung

Videos of acute and chronic mallet fractures, distal phalanx fractures with nail injuries, and early protected movement of K-wired fractures accompany this article

This article discusses unstable finger fractures that require internal fixation to achieve bony stability and joint congruity. The article explains the value of minimally invasive closed reduction and K-wire fixation for the treatment of phalangeal fractures, as well as early protected movement for these K wired fingers, following the concept of early protected movement for flexor tendon repairs.

Minimally Invasive Treatment of Raynaud Phenomenon: The Role of Botulinum Type A 17

Michael W. Neumeister, Kelli Nicole Belangee Webb, and Michael Romanelli

Although the mechanism is unknown, botulinum toxin type A injection may be an effective, localized, nonsurgical treatment option without addictive properties or systemic side effects for the treatment of ischemic digits. Clinical research supports the safety and efficacy of injection of botulinum toxin type A for the treatment of Raynaud phenomenon.

Collagenase Injections for Treatment of Dupuytren Disease 25

Vincent R. Hentz

Dupuytren disease (DD) is a benign, generally painless connective tissue disorder affecting the palmar fascia that leads to progressive hand contractures. Surgical intervention traditionally has been the most effective and widely accepted treatment of progressive contracture. Injection of bacterial derived collagenase into contracting fascial cords emerged as a potential therapeutic option for DD in 1996, offering a potential advantage of target specificity. After rigid clinical trials, collagenase was released by the Food and Drug Administration in 2010 and continues to be studied. Early experience indicates that collagenase fasciotomy is initially equally successful as needle aponeurotomy and its effectiveness seems more durable.

Needle Aponeurotomy for the Treatment of Dupuytren's Disease **33**

Roberto Diaz and Catherine Curtin

Videos of a needle being inserted into an abductor digiti minimi cord and manipulation of a pretendinous cord accompany this article

Surgical treatment of Dupuytren disease includes radical fasciectomy, limited fasciectomy, percutaneous needle aponeurotomy (PNA), and treatment with collagenase injections. The most commonly performed procedure is limited fasciectomy. However, techniques such as PNA and collagenase injections are being performed with higher frequency because they are minimally invasive. PNA is generally recommended for older patients with less severe contractures who desire a faster recovery with a low complication rate. Patients undergoing PNA should be informed that recurrence rates appear to be higher with PNA in comparison with limited fasciectomy.

Percutaneous Release of Trigger Fingers **39**

Edson Sasahara Sato, João Baptista Gomes dos Santos, João Carlos Belloti, Walter Manna Albertoni, and Flavio Faloppa

Minimally invasive approaches to hand problems include the percutaneous treatment of symptomatic trigger fingers. A percutaneous approach allows for an office-based procedure requiring minimal rehabilitation. In a prior study, the authors compared the effectiveness of percutaneous pulley release with corticosteroid and conventional open surgery for treating trigger finger. The percutaneous and open methods displayed similar effectiveness, and both procedures were superior to corticosteroid injection for both cure and relapse rates of trigger finger. The percutaneous method is a safe, minimally invasive alternative for the treatment of trigger fingers.

Endoscopic Carpal Tunnel Release **47**

Torben B. Hansen and Haider Ghalib Majeed

Endoscopic carpal tunnel release is a minimally invasive surgical treatment of carpal tunnel syndrome, which may be performed under local anesthesia and provides a rapid recovery without increasing the risk of complications. After the initial 3 months, no major difference in results has been found compared with open surgery. The endoscopic technique has a significant learning curve and the cost of the operation is higher than with the conventional open technique. However, the faster rehabilitation and the probability of a faster return to work may lead to a more cost-effective patient path compared with conventional open carpal tunnel release.

Endoscopic Release of the Cubital Tunnel **55**

Horst Zajonc and Arash Momeni

Minimally invasive surgery is becoming part of the practice of hand surgery, which includes the adoption of endoscopic techniques for the treatment of cubital tunnel syndrome. Endoscopic cubital tunnel release allows for the advantages of minimal skin incisions and the low morbidity of an in situ release as well as full release of the nerve over a long distance. The authors have used this technique with great success and discuss the procedure, its indications, and outcomes.

Minimal-Incision In Situ Ulnar Nerve Decompression at the Elbow **63**

Joshua M. Adkinson and Kevin C. Chung

A wide variety of surgical techniques are available to treat cubital tunnel syndrome. With expanding evidence for the safety, efficacy, and lower complication profile of in situ cubital tunnel release, the role of this technique has been increasingly defined. The technical modification of minimal-incision–open cubital tunnel release is summarized, highlighting key technical points as well as outcomes studies.

Arthroscopic Excision of Ganglion Cysts **71**

Nicholas A. Bontempo and Arnold-Peter C. Weiss

Dorsal ganglions are benign soft tissue tumors that arise from the scapholunate ligament. If the cyst is creating symptoms of pain, weakness, or difficulty with activity, then surgical excision should be considered. Surgical excision has typically been performed in an open fashion; but over the years, arthroscopy has been adapted as a tool for excision. Although randomized controlled trials are lacking, evidence suggests that arthroscopic excision results in few complications and in recurrence rates that are equal to, if not lower than, open excision. Proposed benefits of arthroscopic excision include improved cosmesis, quicker recovery, and earlier return to work.

Minimally Invasive Approaches to Ulnar-Sided Wrist Disorders **77**

Joseph M. Pirolo and Jeffrey Yao

Ulnar-sided wrist pain is a common cause of upper-extremity disability, which has long been thought of as a diagnostic and therapeutic dilemma because of the overlapping anatomy and complex differential diagnosis. Common sources of ulnar-sided pain include pathology of the triangular fibrocartilage complex, ulnocarpal impaction syndrome, lunotriquetral ligament tears, and hamate arthrosis. The authors discuss the evaluation of these common pathologic conditions and arthroscopic treatment options, including debridement, capsulorrhaphy, ligament repair, osteochondroplasty, microfracture, and arthroscopically assisted percutaneous fixation.

Use of Arthroscopy for the Treatment of Scaphoid Fractures **91**

David J. Slutsky

Scaphoid fractures can be treated with minimal soft tissue dissection using percutaneous methods. Arthroscopy is a helpful tool when using these percutaneous scaphoid screw insertion techniques. Arthroscopy aids in optimal guidewire positioning, it is invaluable in assessing the quality of fracture reduction, and it allows one to evaluate the vascularity of the fracture fragments as well as the stability of fixation. Arthroscopy also allows assessment of screw length ensuring no radiocarpal penetration with retrograde (volar) insertion as well as checking for well-buried screw threads in the proximal pole with dorsal (antegrade) insertion.

Index **105**

HAND CLINICS

FORTHCOMING ISSUES

May 2014
Reconstruction of the Traumatized Upper Extremity
Kevin C. Chung, MD, *Editor*

August 2014
Evidence-based Hand Surgery
Jennifer Waljee, MD and
Kate Nellans, MD, *Editors*

November 2014
Options for Surgical Exposure and Soft Tissue Coverage in Upper Extremity\Trauma
Amitava Gupta MD, FRCS, *Editor*

RECENT ISSUES

November 2013
Management of Hand Fractures
Jeffrey N. Lawton, MD, *Editor*

August 2013
Peripheral Nerve Conditions: Using Evidence to Guide Treatment
Warren C. Hammert, MD, *Editor*

May 2013
Tendon Repair and Reconstruction
Jin Bo Tang, MD, and
Steve K. Lee, MD, *Editors*

February 2013
Anthroplasty Around the Wrist: CMC, Radiocarpal, DRUJ
Kevin C. Chung, MD, *Editor*

Preface

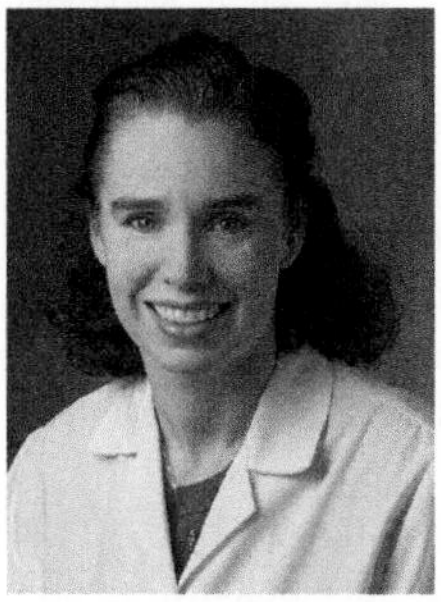

Catherine Curtin, MD
Editor

Minimally invasive surgery is an area of intense interest for both patients and surgeons. Other surgical disciplines have been revolutionized by smaller incisions and exposures. For example, vascular surgery has embraced endovascular techniques, which had previously been performed mainly by interventional radiologists. Now vascular *surgical* residencies include endovascular rotations. Minimal techniques have had a more moderate impact on the field of hand surgery. Hand surgery generally does not require explorations of deep dark holes and thus smaller exposures are common practice. Yet there are still opportunities to reduce soft tissue exposures in hand surgery. Also it is likely that we can reduce overall surgical costs to the patient and the health care system using a minimally invasive surgical approach. This issue provides an overview of the areas where minimally invasive techniques can be incorporated into the practice of hand surgery.

Before reading this issue, a hand surgeon may ask: "why bother with minimally invasive approaches in hand surgery? Our current practice provides safe and effective care." There are several reasons for the hand surgeon to be familiar with these techniques. One primary reason is patient demand. If a surgery can be done as safely and effectively with a smaller incision, then patients will seek out this care. In the emerging health care system, patient preference and satisfaction will take on increasing importance to the practicing hand surgeon. For elective procedures, patients are increasingly using the Internet when choosing a physician and they will seek out the surgeon who can offer a smaller "scar."[1,2] In addition, patient satisfaction is becoming tied to reimbursement. In 2012 Medicare began linking financial incentives to patient satisfaction measures, and smaller surgical exposures are almost always associated with greater patient acceptance.

A second reason supporting the adoption of minimally invasive surgery is the potential impact on costs. Some minimally invasive techniques use less manpower and equipment than alternative methods. Dr Lalonde has shown that his surgery on wide-awake patients can be performed safely with lower use of health care resources. His patients have hand surgery with local anesthetic and often simple field sterility.[3] Cost comparisons have not been widely undertaken on different techniques. Dr Chung performed a study on Dupuytren's treatment and found that percutaneous needle aponeurotomy was more cost effective than collagenase or fasciectomy.[4] Minimally invasive techniques may become more prominent as insurance companies demand the most cost-effective treatments. Minimally invasive procedures not only are procedures with smaller incisions but also have the potential to significantly lower overall costs.

Patient preference and pursuit of the most economic care should not compel us to perform unsafe operations. This issue will detail minimally invasive hand surgery techniques: how they are done and their outcomes. Some of these procedures have been around for decades, such as endoscopic carpal tunnel; others are new approaches to old problems (Dr Lalonde's wide-awake fracture treatment), and some are treatments that have not been widely adopted (percutaneous trigger release). We hope that this presentation of minimally invasive options

Hand Clin 30 (2014) ix–x
http://dx.doi.org/10.1016/j.hcl.2013.09.007
0749-0712/14/$ – see front matter Published by Elsevier Inc.

and their outcomes will help surgeons choose what techniques might safely fit into their practice.

Catherine Curtin, MD
Department of Plastic Surgery
Palo Alto Veterans Hospital
3801 Miranda Avenue
Palo Alto, CA 94304, USA

E-mail address:
curtincatherine@yahoo.com

REFERENCES

1. Emmert M, Meier F, Pisch F, et al. Physician choice making and characteristics associated with using physician-rating websites: cross-sectional study. J Med Internet Res 2013;15(8):e187.
2. Kline AJ, Anderson RB, Davis WH, et al. Minimally invasive technique versus an extensile lateral approach for intra-articular calcaneal fractures. Foot Ankle Int 2013;34(6):773–80.
3. Leblanc MR, Lalonde DH, Thoma A, et al. Is main operating room sterility really necessary in carpal tunnel surgery? A multicenter prospective study of minor procedure room field sterility surgery. Hand (NY) 2011;6(1):60–3.
4. Chen NC, Shauver MJ, Chung KC. Cost-effectiveness of open partial fasciectomy, needle aponeurotomy, and collagenase injection for dupuytren contracture. J Hand Surg Am 2011;36(11):1826–34.

Minimally Invasive Anesthesia in Wide Awake Hand Surgery

Don Lalonde, MD, MSc, FRCSC

KEYWORDS

• Wide-awake • Epinephrine finger • WALANT • Tourniquet-free • Sedation-free

KEY POINTS

- The tourniquet is no longer required for hand surgery because of epinephrine hemostasis.
- Epinephrine in the finger is safe.
- Epinephrine vasoconstriction in the finger is reversible with phentolamine.
- Wide-awake flexor tendon repair has decreased tenolysis and rupture rates.
- Patients like the sedation-free approach for carpal tunnel and find it similar to dental surgery.

Videos of how to inject carpal tunnel with minimal pain for wide awake surgery; Field sterility for surgery; surgery; intraoperative patient advice; bandage; and typical patient impression after surgery accompany this article at http://www.hand.theclinics.com/

INTRODUCTION/NATURE OF THE PROBLEM

One of the most significant recent advances in hand surgery has been the movement away from tourniquet surgery, which often requires sedation or general anesthesia. The advent of epinephrine safety in the finger has led many to use this mode of hemostasis. This is providing a patient experience similar to a visit to the dentist; the patient comes in, rolls up his sleeve, gets the local anesthesia, has the hand surgery and goes home without preoperative testing or postoperative recovery time in the hospital or surgery center.

WHAT IS MINIMALLY INVASIVE ANESTHESIA FOR WIDE-AWAKE HAND SURGERY?

In wide-awake hand surgery, the only medications given to the patient are subcutaneous lidocaine and epinephrine. This mixture is infiltrated wherever surgical dissection, K wire insertion, or manipulation of fractured bones will occur. The concept behind this technique is that the local anesthetic results in an extravascular Bier block but only where it is needed. The other term that is frequently used to describe this approach is tumescent local anesthesia.

There are several advantages to this minimally invasive technique. If the local anesthesia is administered properly,[1] all that the patient feels is the first needle poke of a 27-gauge needle in the hand for most hand operations. The lack of any sedation means there is no need for preoperative testing, intravenous insertion, intraoperative monitoring, or the postoperative anesthetic care unit. The procedures can be performed without sedation, because epinephrine is used for hemostasis, which obviates the need of a painful tourniquet. Once exposed to this concept, the patients love it.[2] The patient experience of hand surgery using this technique becomes more on par with a visit to the dentist.

Surgery, Dalhousie University, Hilyard Place, Suite C204, 600 Main Street, Saint John, New Brunswick E2K 1J5, Canada
E-mail address: drdonlalonde@nb.aibn.com

Hand Clin 30 (2014) 1–6
http://dx.doi.org/10.1016/j.hcl.2013.08.015
0749-0712/14/$ – see front matter

INDICATIONS/CONTRAINDICATIONS

The author and colleagues believe that nearly every patient should be offered the wide-awake option. Most people who do not want sedation at the dentist are likely to prefer the wide-awake approach, because it is more convenient than going through the time-consuming process associated with sedation: preoperative testing, intravenous insertion, and postsedation recovery period. Patients with pre-existing medical problems such as renal dialysis, morbid obesity, and severe lung problems should be considered for this approach, as it is safer than the sedation/general anesthesia route.

Of course, some patients really are better served having sedation, and it should be given to them. Patients with high anxiety or severe post-traumatic stress disorder may not tolerate a wide-awake procedure. Also take care in offering this technique to non-native English speakers and those with cognitive impairments. Finally, not all surgeons enjoy interactive discussion with patients that can occur during operative procedures. This technique is not for those surgeons.

Epinephrine-induced cardiac ischemia is a possible but extremely rare event; even with high doses (1:1000 epinephrine).[3] The author and colleagues have not had this complication with over 2000 cases. However, if there is concern with epinephrine use because of cardiac disease, lowering the dose of epinephrine to 1:400,000 is an option the author and colleagues occasionally employ. Some have even found epinephrine 1:1,000,000 effective for hemostasis.[4]

TECHNIQUE

Anesthetic

It has been shown in liposuction patients that up 35 mg/kg of tumescent lidocaine with epinephrine injection can result in safe blood levels of lidocaine.[5] Nevertheless, the author and colleagues use the conservative upper limit of 7 mg/kg of lidocaine with epinephrine, as their patients are not monitored. In a 70 kg person, this means 49 cc of 1% lidocaine with 1:100,000 epinephrine.

For standard exposures, the author and colleagues inject up to 50 cc of subcutaneous 1% lidocaine with 1:100,000 epinephrine wherever surgical dissection, manipulation of fractured bones, or K wire insertion will occur. If a larger field needs to be anesthetized such as for larger operations such as spaghetti wrist or tendon transfer, the author and colleagues add up to 150 cc of saline to obtain more volume. This results in 0.25% lidocaine with 1:400,000, which is still effective for local anesthesia and hemostasis. However, this dilution does require a little longer to set up.[6] Even 1 in a million epinephrine provides effective hemostasis if a patient has a greatly unstable heart.[4]

For operations longer than 2 hours, the author and colleagues add up to 10 cc of 0.5% bupivacaine with 1:200,000 epinephrine to the infiltrate to make sure no top ups are required. The author and colleagues consider top ups to be a failure of the initial injection, and they should be avoided.

Anesthetic Technique

Patients are placed supine and injected in the holding area before entering the operating room. For this technique to be maximally effective, time must be allowed to let the medication take effect. It has been shown that maximal vasoconstriction occurs an average of 26 minutes after injection of 1:100,000 epinephrine beneath human skin.[7]

For short procedures, the patients are instructed at the time of the preoperative consultation that they should bring a book, as they will have to wait at least 30 minutes between the injection of the local anesthesia and the surgery. They are given the analogy of: "putting a cake in the oven and giving it time to bake." The author and colleagues have developed a system to allow for efficient throughput in their surgical center. Their first 3 patients arrive at 8 AM; the surgeon completes their injection and paperwork. It takes an average of 5 minutes to inject a carpal tunnel patient in a consistently almost pain-free manner.[8] While the third patient is being injected, the nurse sets up the first patient in the operating room. After the first case, the nurse brings the second patient into the operating room and sets it up while the surgeon injects the fourth patient, and so on.

More thought is required when injecting larger areas such as multiple flexor tendons in the hand or for forearm cases. The key to success is that enough volume is injected into the most proximal area to be dissected so that the tissues become mildly indurated or blanched with local anesthesia.[9] Care must be taken when injecting near the nerves; eliciting paresthesias is unnecessary, as tumescent local anesthesia is effective without placing the needle so close to the nerve. In addition, the sharp bevel of the needle can lacerate nerve fascicles. With this technique, the local is injected 5 to 10 mm away from major nerves. Then time is given to allow diffusion of the local to the big nerves while epinephrine vasoconstriction sets in. After injection, there should be at least 1 cm of visible or palpable subcutaneous local anesthesia beyond any area of intended dissection.

Attached are several videos that show the use of this technique for an open carpal tunnel release (Videos 1–6).

HOW TO INJECT MINIMAL PAIN LOCAL ANESTHESIA FOR WIDE-AWAKE HAND SURGERY

There are 2 ways to inject local anesthesia; the traditional method of rapid injection with a 25-gauge needle, or the less painful "blow slow before you go" technique, which hurts patients less. Nine principles of minimal pain local anesthesia are listed in **Box 1**, the details of which have been published elsewhere.[10]

SPECIFIC AREAS OF IMPACT FOR WIDE-AWAKE ANESTHESIA

Flexor Tendon Repair

The wide-awake approach has had an impact on reducing rupture and tenolysis rates after flexor tendon repair.[12–14] There are 4 main reasons for this.

First, after each suture, the repair can be tested with full active flexion and extension by the comfortable, cooperative, unsedated, tourniquet-free patient. This allows the surgeon to assess for gapping generated by sutures that are too loose, which will increase risk of rupture. Thus the surgeon can repair the gap before the skin is closed instead of going on to rupture.

Second, the full active flexion and extension shows the surgeon that the repair fits through the pulleys with active movement. If it does not, pulleys can be vented, or repairs can be trimmed or narrowed with sutures. The entire A2 pulley and up to half of the A4 pulley can be divided if necessary. As the surgeon is observing the active movement, only the pulley that needs to be divided is sacrificed.

Third, the tendon can be repaired inside the sheath, with the needles being introduced through sheathotomy incisions that can be repaired at the end of the case. The reason this is possible is that the patient will demonstrate to the surgeon with full active movement that the inside of the sheath has not been caught by the needle and thread.

Finally, if the surgeon sees the patient making a full fist and extending the fingers completely during the surgery, he or she knows that the patient can be allowed to perform true active early protected movement with half a fist after surgery, as opposed to place and hold. The author and colleagues allow patients to make half a fist and 45° active flexion and extension of each of the MP, PIP, and DIP joints beginning 3 to 5 days after surgery.[15] This is the "half a fist/45/45/45" regime.

Box 1
Methods of decreasing the pain of local anesthetic injection

Step 1. Buffering lidocaine and epinephrine 10:1 with 8.4% bicarbonate[11]

Step 2. Warming the local anesthetic

Step 3. Distracting the patient or the area of injection with touch, pressure, pinching, or ice

Step 4. Using a 27-gauge needle

Step 5. Stabilizing the syringe to avoid needle wobble

Step 6. Injecting 0.5 cc perpendicularly subdermally and pausing until the patient says the needle pain is gone

Step 7. Injecting an additional 2 cc before moving the needle, and then moving antegrade very slowly with 1 cm of local anesthetic always palpable or visible ahead of the needle

Step 8. Reinserting needles within 1 cm of blanched areas

Step 9. Learning from all patients by asking them to score the number of times they felt pain during the injection

Tendon Transfer

One of the most difficult aspects of tendon transfer has been setting the tension of the transfer so it is not too tight or too loose. All surgeons who have done enough transfers understand this.

The ability to watch the comfortable tourniquet-free awake patient flex and extend the involved digits allows for adjustments to be made to the tension before the skin is closed. This technique has taken some of the guesswork out and has improved tensioning during tendon transfer surgery.[16]

Fracture Treatment

Wide-awake surgery for fracture treatment has several advantages. This technique provides intraoperative assessment of full active movement under low-power C arm fluoroscopy. This motion will demonstrate any malrotation that may be present. The ranging of the fingers also allows the surgeon to see any movement in fracture fragments with active finger flexion and extension. Thus the surgeon can ensure adequate K wire stability is achieved to permit early controlled active movement. The technique for wide-awake fracture treatment is outlined in the article by Gregory and colleagues elsewhere in this issue.

COMPLICATIONS/SAFETY

The "Jitters" and Fainting

There are 2 relatively common problems with tumescent lidocaine and epinephrine injection for wide-awake hand surgery. They are easily dealt with if the surgeon is expecting them and takes defensive action.

The first is the nervous jitter or trembling that can accompany epinephrine injection in anyone. It is wise to forewarn all patients after injection that they may end up feeling a little jittery or shaky after the injection similar to the feeling after consuming too much coffee. The author and colleagues counsel the patient that this is a normal reaction to the adrenaline in the numbing medicine; that the feeling will go away all by itself in 20 to 30 minutes, and that this is not an allergic reaction to the local anesthetic.

The second common problem is a vasovagal episode.[17] This occurs when there is not enough blood going to the brain.[18] The vasovagal response is limited by injecting patients lying down instead of sitting up. Even lying down, some patients may complain that they are not feeling well or that they are going to be sick. They may also get pale between the eyes or in the glabella. These are all signs of imminent fainting, and they are best treated by flexing the hips and knees to get thigh blood to the brain quickly. The head pillow can be removed and placed under the feet. The stretcher can be placed in the Trendelenberg position (head down and feet up). These measures will have the patients feeling much better in a matter of minutes.

Safety of Epinephrine in the Finger

The safety of epinephrine in the finger is now well established.[19,20] The myth of epinephrine danger was generated in the first half of the 20th century when fingers were lost due to procaine acidity.[21] Epinephrine causes vasoconstriction in the human finger, but there is an antidote to this effect: phentolamine. The white finger can be reversed by subcutaneous injection of 1 mg of phentolamine in 2 20 cc of saline wherever the epinephrine is injected.[22] In reality, most fingertips still have good perfusion even when the proximal finger has vasoconstriction, so phentolamine is rarely required in clinical practice. However, if the fingertip should have poor refill and it is time for patient discharge, the vasoconstriction can be reversed.

There are still no cases of finger death associated with accidental finger injection of high-dose (1:1000) epinephrine in spite of hundreds of case reports.[23,24] Patients who have poor perfusion to fingertips with slow refill before the surgery should likely not have epinephrine in the finger. However, if there is good perfusion in the fingertip before the surgery, there will likely be good perfusion after the surgery unless the surgeon damages the blood flow with his or her dissection.

Safety of No Monitoring for Wide-Awake Hand Surgery

Injecting lidocaine with epinephrine is safe. For more than 60 years, in the developed world, millions of injections of lidocaine with epinephrine have been administered safely without monitoring in dental offices.[25,26] Most Mohs surgeons do not monitor vital signs in patients who have skin cancers removed, and this practice has been reported to be safe.[27] Everywhere throughout the world, other minor procedures are performed with lidocaine anesthesia without monitoring on a regular basis with only rare adverse reactions reported. The severe adverse reactions of anaphylaxis to lidocaine are extremely rare.[28–31]

Preoperative assessment and intraoperative monitoring are the norm in North America when sedation is given to patients. The issue is about the sedation and not the local anesthesia or the surgery itself.

OUTCOMES

Patient Satisfaction

There is a popular misconception by many that patients need sedation for minor hand operations such as carpal tunnel surgery. In fact, it has been shown that carpal tunnel patient satisfaction with local anesthetic is high for surgery with or without sedation.[17,32] There is level 3 evidence that patients will choose the anesthetic technique recommended by their surgeon and have equal satisfaction.[2]

Patient satisfaction is high with wide-awake minor procedures such as carpal tunnel surgery and trigger finger release, because the experience is even less cumbersome than a dental visit. The hand surgeon is not operating in the mouth, and patients just hold out their hand for the surgery and do not need to watch. Yet the same in-and-out of the office convenience of dental surgery remains. The tourniquet pain of brief carpal tunnel surgery is twice the pain of the injection of local anesthesia with epinephrine for hemostasis (level 3 evidence).[33] Using epinephrine avoids tourniquet discomfort.

Patients do not have the postoperative nausea and vomiting associated with sedation and narcotic administration. They do not have to take time out of work or get a baby sitter so they can go for preoperative blood work (another needle), chest radiographs or electrocardiograms. Patients spend far less time at the hospital the day they have their surgery[2] and require no special precautions related to the sedation after the surgery.

Surgeon Satisfaction and Cost Implications

Removing the need for sedation and the tourniquet removes the need for minor hand surgery to be performed in the setting of the main operating room. Carpal tunnel surgery can be performed with field sterility in the minor procedure room of a clinic or office with the same low infection rate and full sterility of the main operating room.[34] Field sterility means that the masked and gloved surgeon does not wear a gown and only uses towel to drape the hand.[35]

Three carpal tunnels/trigger fingers per hour can be performed in the clinic or office setting with just 1 nurse to help the surgeon.[36] The cost improvements for the surgeon operating in the private sector are massive.[37]

In addition to the greatly decreased expense of the surgery, the surgeon does not need to worry about wasted turnover time. While the nurse turns over the room and brings in the next patient, the surgeon can go and inject the local anesthesia in a waiting patient in the preoperative holding area. By the time he has done that, the next patient in the operating room is ready for surgery.

Talking to the unsedated patient during the surgery has many benefits. The personal touch could potentially reduce lawsuit risk. Discussions about return to activities and work can happen while the surgeon is working. Learning a little about the patient can lead to postoperative management advice that can decrease complication risks, which further improves time management for the surgeon.

SUMMARY

Tumescent minimally invasive local anesthesia is eliminating the need for sedation and proximal nerve blocks as well as all of their risks, costs, and inconveniences. It has facilitated advances in procedures such as hand fracture reduction, tendon repair, and tendon transfer by allowing the surgeon to see cooperative patient active movement during the surgery. It has improved the patient experience for simple hand operations such as carpal tunnel release.

SUPPLEMENTARY DATA

Supplementary data related to this article can be found online at http://dx.doi.org/10.1016/j.hcl.2013.08.015.

REFERENCES

1. Farhangkhoee H, Lalonde J, Lalonde DH. Teaching medical students and residents how to inject local anesthesia almost painlessly. Can J Plast Surg 2012;20(3):169.
2. Davison PG, Cobb T, Lalonde DH. The patient's perspective on carpal tunnel surgery related to the type of anesthesia: a prospective cohort study. Hand (N Y) 2013;8:47.
3. Cunnington C, McDonald JE, Singh RK. Epinephrine-induced myocardial infarction in severe anaphylaxis: is nonselective β-blockade a contributory factor? J Emerg Med 2013;31(4):759.e1–2.
4. Prasetyono TO. Tourniquet-free hand surgery using the one-per-mil tumescent technique. Arch Plast Surg 2013;40(2):129–33.
5. Burk RW 3rd, Guzman-Stein G, Vasconez LO. Lidocaine and epinephrine levels in tumescent technique liposuction. Plast Reconstr Surg 1996;97(7):1379–84.
6. Mustoe TA, Buck DW II, Lalonde DH. The safe management of anesthesia, sedation and pain in plastic surgery. Plast Reconstr Surg 2010;126(4):165e–76e.
7. McKee DE, Lalonde DH, Thoma A, et al. Optimal time delay between epinephrine injection and incision to minimize bleeding. Plast Reconstr Surg 2013;131(4):811.
8. Lalonde DH. "Hole-in-one" local anesthesia for wide awake carpal tunnel surgery. Plast Reconstr Surg 2010;126(5):1642.
9. Lalonde DH. Reconstruction of the hand with wide awake surgery. Clin Plast Surg 2011;38(4):761–9.
10. Strazar AR, Leynes PG, Lalonde DH. Minimizing the pain of local anesthesia injection. Plast Reconstr Surg 2013;132(3):675.
11. Frank SG, Lalonde DH. How acidic is the lidocaine we are injecting, and how much bicarbonate should we add? Can J Plast Surg 2012;20(2):71.
12. Higgins A, Lalonde DH, Bell M, et al. Avoiding flexor tendon repair rupture with intraoperative total active movement examination. Plast Reconstr Surg 2010;126(3):941.
13. Lalonde DH, Kozin S. Tendon disorders of the hand. Plast Reconstr Surg 2011;128(1):1e–14e.
14. Lalonde DH. Wide-awake flexor tendon repair. Plast Reconstr Surg 2009;123(2):623.
15. Lalonde DH. How the wide awake approach is changing hand surgery and hand therapy. J Hand Ther 2013;26(3):175.
16. Bezuhly M, Sparkes GL, Higgins A, et al. Immediate thumb extension following extensor indicis proprius to extensor pollicis longus tendon transfer using the wide awake approach. Plast Reconstr Surg 2007;119(5):1507.
17. Teo I, Lam W, Muthayya P, et al. Patients' perspective of wide-awake hand surgery—100 consecutive cases. J Hand Surg Eur Vol 2013;132(3):675.

18. Raj SR, Coffin ST. Medical therapy and physical maneuvers in the treatment of the vasovagal syncope and orthostatic hypotension. Prog Cardiovasc Dis 2013;55(4):425–33.
19. Mann T. Hammert WC Epinephrine and hand surgery. J Hand Surg Am 2012;37(6):1254–6.
20. Lalonde DH, Bell M, Benoit P, et al. A multicenter prospective study of 3110 consecutive cases of elective epinephrine use in the fingers and hand: the Dalhousie Project clinical phase. J Hand Surg Am 2005;30:1061.
21. Thomson CJ, Lalonde DH, Denkler KA. A critical look at the evidence for and against elective epinephrine use in the finger. Plast Reconstr Surg 2007;119(1):260.
22. Nodwell T, Lalonde DH. How long does it take phentolamine to reverse adrenaline-induced vasoconstriction in the finger and hand? A prospective randomized blinded study: the Dalhousie project experimental phase. Can J Plast Surg 2003;11(4):187.
23. Muck AE, Bebarta VS, Borys DJ, et al. Six years of epinephrine digital injections: absence of significant local or systemic effects. Ann Emerg Med 2010; 56(3):270–4.
24. Fitzcharles-Bowe C, Denkler KA, Lalonde DH. Finger injection with high-dose (1:1000) epinephrine: does it cause finger necrosis and should it be treated? Hand (N Y) 2007;2(1):5.
25. Gaffen AS, Haas DA. Survey of local anesthetic use by Ontario dentists. J Can Dent Assoc 2009;75(9): 649.
26. Jeske AH. Xylocaine: 50 years of clinical service to dentistry. Tex Dent J 1998;115(5):9–13.
27. Larson MJ, Taylor RS. Monitoring vital signs during outpatient Mohs and post-Mohs reconstructive surgery performed under local anesthesia. Dermatol Surg 2004;30(5):777–83.
28. Baluga JC. Allergy to local anesthetics in dentistry. Myth or reality? Rev Alerg Mex 2003;50(5): 176–81.
29. Speca SJ, Boynes SG, Cuddy MA. Allergic reactions to local anesthetic formulations. Dent Clin North Am 2010;54:655–64.
30. Chiu CY, Lin TY, Hsia SH, et al. Systemic anaphylaxis following local lidocaine administration during a dental procedure. Pediatr Emerg Care 2004;20(3): 178–80.
31. Bircher AJ, Surber C. Anaphylactic reaction to lidocaine. Aust Dent J 1999;44(1):64.
32. Koegst WH, Wölfle O, Thoele K, et al. The "wide awake approach" in hand surgery: a comfortable anaesthesia method without a tourniquet. Handchir Mikrochir Plast Chir 2011;43(3):175–80.
33. Braithwaite BD, Robinson GJ, Burge PD. Haemostasis during carpal tunnel release under local anaesthesia: a controlled comparison of a tourniquet and adrenaline infiltration. J Hand Surg Br 1993; 18:184.
34. Leblanc MR, Lalonde DH, Thoma A, et al. Is main operating room sterility really necessary in carpal tunnel surgery? A multicenter prospective study of minor procedure room field sterility surgery. Hand (N Y) 2011;6(1):60–3.
35. Carpal tunnel syndrome; evidence based leading edge MOC. Plas Reconstr Surg, in press.
36. Leblanc MR, Lalonde J, Lalonde DH. A detailed cost and efficiency analysis of performing carpal tunnel surgery in the main operating room versus the ambulatory setting in Canada. Hand (N Y) 2007; 2(4):173.
37. Bismil MS, Bismil QM, Harding D, et al. Transition to total one-stop wide-awake hand surgery service-audit: a retrospective review. JRSM Short Rep 2012;3:23.

Minimally Invasive Finger Fracture Management

Wide-awake Closed Reduction, K-wire Fixation, and Early Protected Movement

Sol Gregory, BHK, MD[a],
Donald H. Lalonde, MD, MSc, FRCSC[b,*],
Leslie Tze Fung Leung, BSc(Pharm), MD[a]

KEYWORDS

• Finger fracture • K wire • Phalanx • Closed reduction

KEY POINTS

- This article explains why closed reduction can lead to superior results compared with open reduction for finger fractures.
- This article introduces the concept of early protected movement after closed reduction and K-wire fixation of finger fractures.
- This article discusses specific operative techniques for closed reduction K-wire fixation of finger fractures.
- This article compares outcomes between open and closed techniques for the management of finger fractures.

Videos of acute and chronic mallet fractures, distal phalanx fractures with nail injuries, and early protected movement of K-wired fractures accompany this article at http://www.heartfailure.theclinics.com/

INTRODUCTION: NATURE OF THE PROBLEM

An open approach to fractures requires substantial soft tissue dissection. A wound is created every time a fracture is treated openly. Within this wound, the gliding tendons and moving joint structures are exposed to the postoperative healing process and ultimately are affected by restrictive scar tissue and callus formation. The blood that fills the surgical wound creates an inflammatory response, adding more scarring and callus. All the foreign materials left in the wound, such as plates, occupy space, hindering tendon and joint movement. In addition, scar always forms over the plate and can be 1 to 2 mm thick. Each of these processes contributes to limitations of tendon and joint mobility.

Despite its negative impact on the soft tissue envelope, open reduction and internal fixation of unstable finger fractures is recommended because it is thought that more rigid fixation (ie, plate or screw) allows early range of motion, thereby preventing adhesions and stiffness. However, fingers differ from other bones in the body with their small size and high mobility demands. The finger's small

Disclosure: The authors have no disclosures.

[a] Department of Plastic Surgery, University of British Columbia, 899 West 12th Avenue, Vancouver, British of Colombia V5Z1M9, Canada; [b] Department of Plastic Surgery, Dalhousie University, Hilyard Place, Suite C204, 600 Main Street, Saint John NB E2K 1J5, Canada
* Corresponding author.
E-mail address: drdonlalonde@nb.aibn.com

Hand Clin 30 (2014) 7–15
http://dx.doi.org/10.1016/j.hcl.2013.08.014

soft tissue envelope and close proximity of gliding structures can cause stiffness and swelling with any soft tissue dissection, negating the advantage of rigid fixation.

A less invasive approach using K wires can overcome some of the problems with an open approach. When a finger is treated with closed reduction and K-wire fixation, the advantage is that there is no scarring from surgical dissection. There is reduced space for postoperative internal bleeding to accumulate and evolve into callus and scar formation. In addition, there is no hardware to restrict motion. K wires also provide functionally stable fixation. Although not rigid, this type of fixation allows bone to heal in a good position of function so that gliding and good range of motion is achieved. K-wire fixation has advantages suited to the unique issues of finger fractures.

The major concern about K-wire fixation for finger fractures is that the fixation is not strong enough to allow early movement. Early protected movement for finger fractures is important because a stiff finger is a useless finger. The concerns that surgeons have traditionally had with regard to early protected movement with K-wire fixated finger fractures are (1) fear of loss of reduction, and (2) skin irritation/infections generated by K wires. We believe that both these concerns can be minimized, allowing the benefits of K wires and early protected motion.

To minimize risk and optimize the results with K-wire fracture fixation, we have developed a protocol that allows early mobilization after K-wire fixation. In the appropriate patient population, this technique uses minimal soft tissue dissection and allows early motion. The technique relies on the patients' perception of pain to ensure that the motion does not exceed the stability of the fracture reduction construct. This article provides an overview of the technique, patient selection, and the postoperative protocol.

INDICATIONS AND CONTRAINDICATIONS

Patient selection is critical for the success of early protected movement after closed reduction and wide-awake K-wire fixation of finger fractures. **Table 1** provides a list of the indications and contraindications.

Table 1
Patient selection: indications and contraindications

Indications	Contraindications
Patient willing to have wide-awake finger fracture surgery	Fracture not amenable to closed reduction with K wires
Cooperative patient off of all pain medication: understands to not move the finger if painful	Fracture fragment movement after K-wire fixation when tested with active patient movement during wide-awake surgery
Fracture amenable to K-wire reduction	Uncooperative patient on pain medication should not be allowed to do early active movement after surgery
Stable reduction of fracture with K wires: confirmed during wide-awake surgery when the patient intraoperatively tests the fixation with active movement	

PREOPERATIVE PLANNING

The wide-awake surgical reduction permits intraoperative patient active movement assessment before and after K-wire closed reduction. Patients are usually cooperative when it is explained to them that surgeons can do a better job if they see the patient move the fracture during the surgery. The surgeon must first clarify the diagnosis of the finger fracture before proceeding with K-wire fixation. Diligent history focusing on the mechanism of injury, thorough clinical examination, and careful review of 3-view radiographs are crucial for understanding the nature of the fracture, including type and location. In addition, patient factors such as occupation, compliance, and handedness should be respected when planning the operation.

Choosing the appropriate technique of K-wire fixation depends on the location and pattern of the fracture and is discussed later. The surgeon should also anticipate the need to convert the operation into open reduction and internal fixation and have the equipment ready.

PREP AND PATIENT POSITIONING

The patient's hand is prepped and sterilized using chlorhexidine solution and placed on a properly draped hand table. A fluoroscopy device needs to be accessible to assess the fracture reduction during the operation. We prefer a low-power device to minimize patient and surgeon radiation dosage. The patient should receive antibiotic prophylaxis before the procedure.

SURGICAL APPROACH

The purpose of K-wire fixation of finger fractures is to achieve a functional and stable reduction, which means that an anatomically perfect reduction is not the goal. However, the reduction needs to be functional, with full range of active motion and no scissoring. The wide-awake approach permits the surgeon to test the stability of the K-wire fixation during the surgery as the cooperative tourniquet-free patient takes the finger through a full active range of motion (see the movie on wide-awake finger fracture reduction in Ref.[1])

PROXIMAL PHALANGEAL SHAFT FRACTURES

Overview

Proximal phalangeal fractures account for most phalangeal fractures of the hand.[2] Percutaneous K-wire fixation offers the theoretic advantages of minimizing soft tissue damage and associated tendon adhesion while allowing early active motion of the proximal interphalangeal joint (PIP).

Operative Technique

In all techniques, reduction of the fracture is usually first achieved by flexion of the metacarpophalangeal (MCP) joints to stop the proximal fragment from moving.[1,3–5] The collateral ligaments tighten when the MCP joint is flexed 90°, thereby providing stability to the proximal fragment. The fracture pattern guides the placement of the K wires. Overall, we try to limit the use of K wires across the joints to minimize postoperative stiffness.

technique selection

Extra-articular technique In the extra-articular approach, a 0.9-mm (0.035-inch) K wire is driven anterogradely either ulnar or radial to the base of the proximal phalanx, avoiding the metacarpal head and the extensor tendon.[5]

A second retrograde K wire is usually driven across the fracture to secure the reduction.[6]

Postoperative active and passive range of motion may be started across all joints with the physiotherapist,[5] but we prefer to wait 2 to 4 days. We keep the hand elevated and tell the patient the hand is on strike until internal bleeding stops, swelling is settled, the patient is off pain medication, but before collagen formation starts on day 3.

Cross K-wire technique In the management of short oblique proximal phalangeal fracture, the cross-pinning technique may be considered. Two anterograde 0.9-mm (0.035-inch) K wires are driven from the ulnar and radial side of the proximal phalanx base and crossed to hug the fracture site in a secure position (**Fig. 1**).

Transverse technique In managing unstable long oblique or spiral fracture of the proximal phalanx, two or three 0.9-mm (0.035-inch) K wires maybe driven perpendicular to the fracture line or to the longitudinal axis of the bone (**Fig. 2**).[1,7]

PIP DORSAL FRACTURE DISLOCATION

Overview

The surgeon must understand the unique properties of the PIP joint. The PIP joint has the greatest range of flexion and even minor reductions in motion can result in significant disability. The goals of fixing PIP joint fracture dislocation are to restore range of motion, maintain joint congruity to avoid pain and arthritis, and to prevent deformities.

The surgeon should take care in technique selection for PIP joint fracture. For dorsally subluxated fractures involving less than 40% of the articular surface, the closed dorsal blocking K-wire approach described later is our preferred technique because it allows early protected movement of all joints and there is little dissection.

For unstable fractures involving more than 40% of the articular surface, dynamic traction splinting devices have been helpful.[8–13] The senior author still prefers a short version of the Schenk banjo

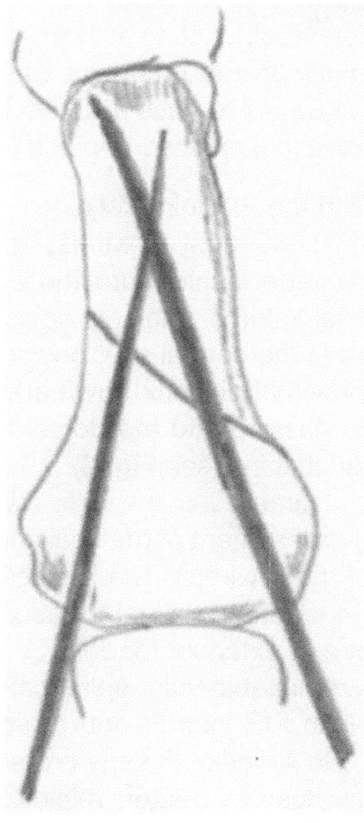

Fig. 1. Cross-pinning technique for proximal phalanx shaft fractures.

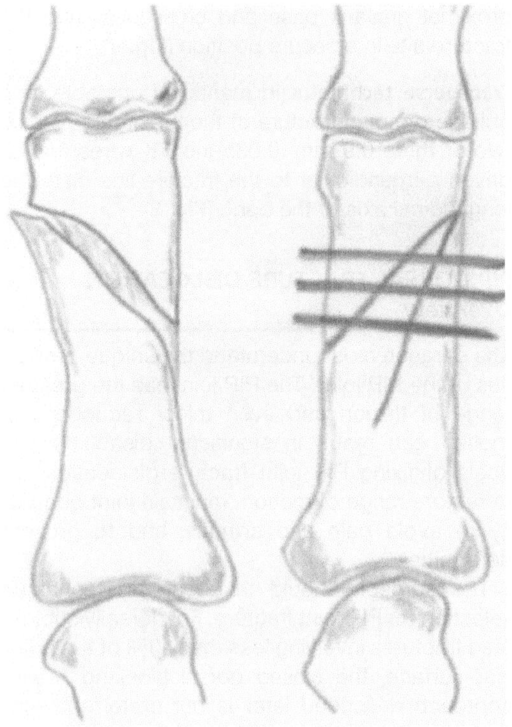

Fig. 2. Transverse K-wire fixation of long oblique fracture of proximal phalanx.

splint, even though he has tried the multiple K-wire techniques, which have not worked as well.

Operative Technique

Dorsal blocking K-wire fixation

Sustained dorsal subluxation of the middle phalanx leads to joint damage and stiffness. One method to manage this injury is to pass a K wire through the PIP joint as a dorsal extensor block (**Fig. 3**).[14]

Step 1: With the PIP joint in flexion, one or two 0.9-mm (0.035-inch) K wire(s) are drilled in the retrograde fashion into the bare area of the dorsal middle phalanx adjacent to the insertion of the central slip, pushing the base of the proximal phalanx down and keeping it there by passing into the dorsal head of the proximal phalanx (see **Fig. 3**).[17]
Active movement with the wide-awake patient permits assessment of the final angle and position of the K wire(s). The K wires should be placed such that minimal irritation occurs to the joint and extensor tendons.

Step 2: A removable volar splint can be placed to maintain PIP joint flexion at about 10° to 30° for 3 to 4 weeks.[15] Early protected movement, as described later, minimize stiffness. K-wire irritation of the skin is minimized when pain guides the patient's activity.

MIDDLE PHALANGEAL SHAFT FRACTURES

Overview

Middle phalangeal fractures are less common than proximal and distal phalanx fractures.[2] There is little literature regarding closed reduction and percutaneous K-wire fixation of unstable middle phalangeal shaft fractures.

Operative Technique

Two techniques are described: anterograde cross-pinning from the base of the middle phalanx or retrograde pinning from the head of the middle phalanx.[1,16]

Step 1: Closed reduction is first achieved by flexing the PIP and the DIP joint at 90 degrees. This maneuver maintains reduction of the fracture through the traction of the collateral ligaments.[17]

Step 2: In the anterograde approach, two 0.7-mm or 0.9-mm (0.028-inch or 0.035-inch) K wires are cross-pinned from the base of the middle phalanx, in a the midcoronal plane, to the subchondral bone of the phalangeal head; in the retrograde approach, the K wires are introduced from the retrocondylar fossa of the middle phalangeal head into the lateral bases of the phalanx. In managing transverse middle phalangeal neck fracture, a single K wire may be passed in a retrograde fashion through the head of the proximal phalanx, and then the wire is driven in an anterograde fashion to free the PIP joint while keeping the DIP joint extended.[17] If possible, we do not leave the K wires across the PIP joint at the end of the procedure, and we try to limit the damage to the articular cartilage from the K-wire passes

Testing the construct with active movement during the surgery determines how many K wires are needed.

DISTAL INTERPHALANGEAL JOINT FRACTURE (BONY MALLET DEFORMITY)

Overview

Avulsion fracture of the base of the dorsal distal phalanx is an injury caused by sudden forced flexion, hyperextension, or longitudinal compression of an extended DIP joint. Most of these injuries can be treated conservatively with splints.

It is frequently written that when more than one-third of the articular surface of the distal phalanx is involved, surgical treatment is indicated to prevent osteoarthritis and stiffness.[18] However, the most important factor affecting the decision to surgically

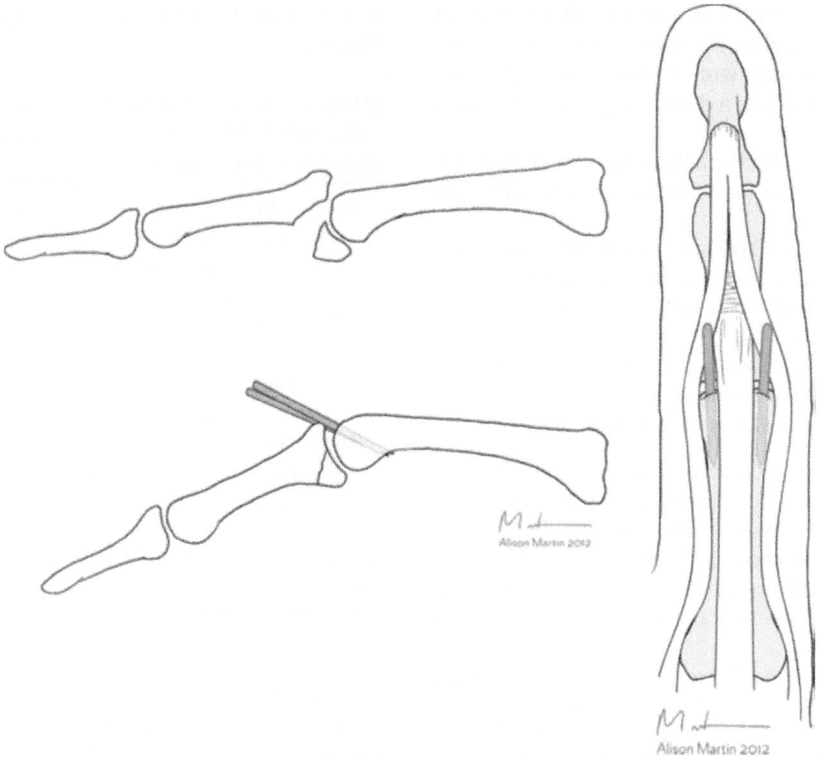

Fig. 3. Dorsal blocking K-wire technique for reducible PIP fracture dislocations. (*Left*) Two dorsal K wires between the central slip and the lateral band reduce the dorsally subluxated middle phalanx (lateral view). (*Right*) Dorsal view. Early protected movement is permitted. (*From* Jones NF, Jupiter JB, Lalonde DH. Common fractures and dislocations of the hand. Plast Reconstr Surg 2012;130:722e–36e; with permission.)

treat a mallet deformity is whether the joint is subluxated. In our experience, fractures with up to 60% of the articular surface can be treated with splinting if the joint is not subluxated. However, we consider that, if the joint is subluxated, surgical closed reduction and K-wire fixation is indicated (Video 1).

Complications of open reduction and internal fixation of this injury may include skin necrosis, nail deformities, extension lag, and infection.[19] Percutaneous K-wire fixation minimizes these complications associated with open procedures.

Operative Technique

Extension blocking K-wire fixation

The authors use the Ishiguro extension blocking K-wire technique[19–21]:

Step 1: Begin by reducing the displaced articular fragment by flexing the DIP and PIP. Flexion of the distal phalanx improves the congruity of the articular surface without volar subluxation; with extension, the fragment is pushed back dorsally (**Fig. 4**).[19]

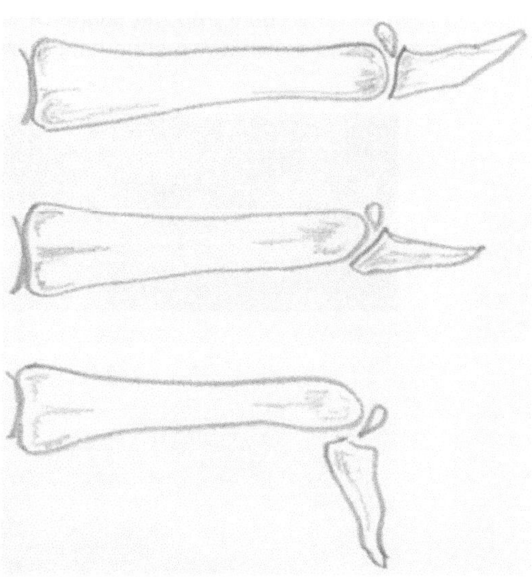

Fig. 4. Reduction of mallet finger is best achieved with DIP flexion. (*Data from* Ishiguro T, Imai N, Tomatsu T, et al. A new method of closed reduction using the spring action of Kirschner wires for fractures of the tibial plateau–a preliminary report. Nihon Seikeigeka Gakkai zasshi 1986;60:227–36.)

Step 2: A 0.7-mm or 0.9-mm (0.028-inch or 0.035-inch) K wire is then inserted 1 to 2 mm above the fragment into the head of the middle phalanx with a dorsal angulation of around 30° to 40°.

Step 3: The distal phalanx is then pulled and pushed up at the volar base to complete the reduction.

Step 4: A second 0.7-mm or 0.9-mm K wire is inserted from the ulnar or the radial side to secure the DIP joint while avoiding the fracture line (**Fig. 5**).

Step 5: The K wires are left in place for 4 to 8 weeks depending on the age of the patient and the circulation of the finger.

The Ishiguro technique has been modified by several investigators with favorable outcomes. Some modifications include using double K wires as the extension block[22] and reducing the fragment at extension by inserting the K wire in a proximal-to-distal direction and pushing the fragment distally.[23]

Badia and Riano[24] insert a 1.1-mm (0.045-inch) K wire from the tip of the distal phalanx across the DIP to keep it at extension; a second K wire is then inserted dorsally to catch the avulsed fragment by acting as a joystick.

The Fanfani umbrella-handle method allows full active motion of the DIP joint immediately after the surgery.[25] In this method, a 1-mm (0.045-inch) K wire is inserted from proximal to distal into the fragment, acting as a joystick. The dorsal, exposed K wire is then bent into the shape of an umbrella handle and drawn down subcutaneously to reduce the fracture while avoiding the DIP joint (**Fig. 6**).

CHRONIC MALLET FRACTURES WITH A VOLARLY SUBLUXATED DISTAL PHALANX

Operative Technique

Step 1: the authors prefer to push dorsally on the volarly subluxated distal phalanx base for several minutes until the joint is reduced by gradual stretching of the DIP collateral ligaments.

Step 2: the DIP joint is then K wired into the reduced position with a 0.9-mm (0.035-inch) K wire without incisions.

Step 3: the K wire is left in place for 8 weeks. The patient is placed in a mallet splint, which enables PIP flexion.

DISTAL PHALANGEAL FRACTURES

Overview

Distal phalangeal fractures are the most common hand fractures, often occurring when the finger is crushed between objects.[26] Nonoperative treatment usually involves protective splinting for 2 to 4 weeks until no longer tender.[27,28]

Operative Techniques

The nail is an exoskeleton to the nail bed and the bone

The nail, the nail bed, and the bone are fixed as 1 unit, so the nail is an exoskeleton to the nail bed and the bone. When the distal phalanx is comminuted but has the nail attached in more

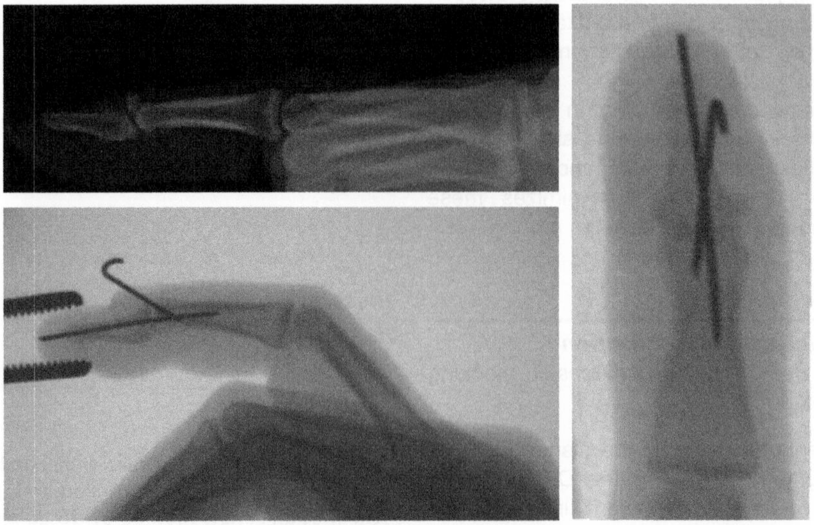

Fig. 5. The Ishiguro technique. (*Data from* Ishiguro T, Imai N, Tomatsu T, et al. A new method of closed reduction using the spring action of Kirschner wires for fractures of the tibial plateau–a preliminary report. Nihon Seikeigeka Gakkai zasshi 1986;60:227–36.)

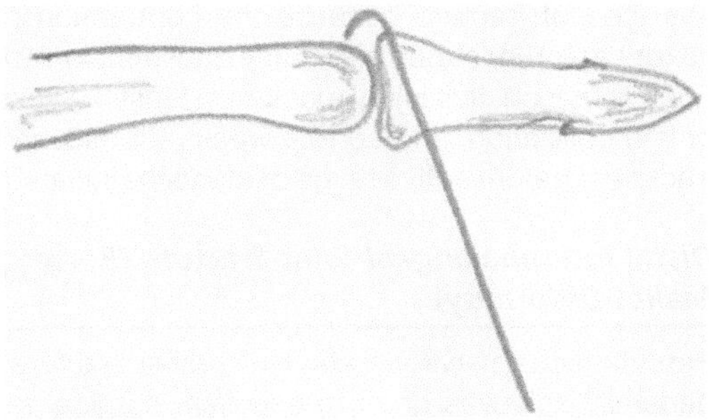

Fig. 6. The Fanfani umbrella-handle technique. (*Data from* Rocchi L, Genitiempo M, Fanfani F. Percutaneous fixation of mallet fractures by the "umbrella handle" technique. J Hand Surg 2006;31:407–12.)

than one fragment, the authors prefer to suture the nail to itself, as in reducing a puzzle. The bigger pieces that can be more easily fixed are sutured first. In so doing, the fragments of nail bed and bone follow the reduced pieces of nail and become reduced (Video 2).

K-wire fixation in distal phalanx fractures

If the bones of the distal phalanx are separated by 2 mm or more and the possibility of nonunion exists, the authors use a 0.7-mm or 0.9-mm (0.028-inch or 0.035-inch) K wire to fixate the fracture in a closed fashion along with mallet splinting for 8 weeks.

COMPLICATIONS AND MANAGEMENT

There are several complications after treatment of K-wire fixation (**Table 2**).

POSTOPERATIVE CARE

After the procedure, the patient's hand is immobilized in a bulky dressing and immobilized in a splint. We counsel the patients that the hand is on strike and it should be elevated above the heart for the first 2 to 4 days until the swelling is gone.

Table 2
Post–K-wire complications and management

Complication	Management
Joint contracture	Splinting Physiotherapy Surgical correction
Stiffness	Physiotherapy
Significant rotational deformities	Surgical correction
Pin site infection	Antibiotics If severe, pin removal (rare)

This time of immobility allows the internal wounds from the K-wire insertion to clot, avoiding further internal bleeding, and allows the pain to improve enough to allow cessation of pain medications. We begin early protected movement only when the patient has stopped all painkillers, including ibuprofen and acetaminophen (usually 2 to 4 days after K wiring). After the discontinuation of pain medications, the patient is allowed to gently move the finger while stabilizing the fracture with the fingers of the other hand. This gentle movement is predicated on the following instruction: do not do anything that hurts. The patient needs to keep the joints moving enough so the tendons and joints do not get stuck. Even a small amount of movement keeps the joints and tendons gliding. The guiding principle of this technique is that the patient lets the pain of the fracture and K-wire skin irritation be the rehabilitation guide.

When patients are completely off all analgesics, they are allowed to move the finger but not allowed to use it (Video 3). If they do something that hurts significantly, they should not try that movement again for 2 to 3 days. The hand is splinted at all times when not doing early protected movement. We allow early active movement every hour while awake and when convenient. When it no longer hurts to move it, they can use it. Clinicians say, "Don't baby it but don't do what hurts" to explain this concept to patients.

The K wires are generally left in place for an average of 2 to 3 weeks. However, when the fracture is not tender to firm palpation between a thumb and index finger, the K wires can usually be removed; this is a clinically healed fracture. Radiological healing lags behind clinical healing for finger fractures and should not be used as a main guide.

The risk of clinically significant loss of fracture reduction with this protocol has been lower than the risk of tendon rupture in early protected movement with flexor tendon repair in our experience, and easier to rectify. K-wire irritation of skin is minimal if the patient pays attention to the pain. We tell them: "We didn't spend 2 billion years evolving pain because it is bad for us! It is nature's only way for our bodies to tell us: 'Hey, stop that! I'm trying to heal in here and you are messing it up!' You can't hear that little voice in your head if you have ibuprofen or acetaminophen in your ears." Most reasonable patients understand this and think that it makes sense.

OUTCOMES

Proximal Phalangeal Fractures

In a prospective case series of 100 displaced, transverse proximal phalangeal fractures, Belsky and colleagues[3] first reported good to excellent functional outcomes in patients who underwent K-wire fixation using the transmetacarpal approach. Subsequent smaller, retrospective case series also showed favorable mean total active motions in most patients.[29,30]

More recently, Faruqui and colleagues[5] compared the transmetacarpal approach with the cross-pinning technique and the total active motions in both groups were comparable. In contrast, in a subgroup retrospective analysis of 49 transverse proximal phalangeal fractures, Al-Qattan[31] reported better total active motion scores in the extra-articular technique versus the transmetacarpal approach in an earlier study. Overall, there are no obvious differences in functional outcomes between percutaneous K-wire fixation and open reduction internal fixation of proximal phalangeal fractures.[6,7,32]

PIP Dorsal Fracture Dislocation

Trans-articular dorsal extensor block with K wire has been shown to produce less deformity and increased range of motion compared with open procedures in 1 prospective study.[33] A long-term study shows that this method achieves satisfactory functional outcomes with only minor degenerative changes at 16-year follow up.[14]

Ikeda and colleagues[34] described a more technically demanding K-wire fixation technique with satisfactory results. In their study, a 1.2-mm (0.047 inch) K wire is inserted as a flexion blocking pin with the PIP joint hyperextended to achieve reduction. Three subsequent K wires are inserted interfragmentarily to maintain final fixation before the flexion blocking pin is removed. The patient is then splinted in full extension for 4 weeks.

The prognosis of PIP fracture dislocation depends on the percentage of articular surface involved and the congruency of the joint following fixation. It is necessary to have a fine balance between allowing the injury to heal and avoiding prolonged immobilization, which results in contracture and stiffness. There is currently no consensus in the literature on the optimal timing on postoperative mobilization. However, most investigators have advocated for passive[35] or active[1,15] range of flexion of the PIP joint immediately after extension blocking K-wire fixation.

Middle Phalangeal Fracture

Postoperative outcomes and rehabilitation regimens following K-wire fixation of middle phalangeal fractures are based on expert opinion, because there are no published data addressing this area. Early active motion may be risky for this type of fracture because the contraction of flexor digitorum superficialis may cause malunion. For this reason, this injury requires at least 3 weeks of immobilization, and up to 6 weeks for midshaft fractures, before active range of motion is initiated.

Distal Interphalangeal Joint Fracture (Bony Mallet Deformity)

Percutaneous K-wire fixation of mallet fractures generally achieves good to excellent surgical results with up to 10° extension lag, full flexion, and no pain according to Crawford's[36] criteria.[15,20–25] These procedures permit the patient to have active range of motion of the metacarpophalangeal joint and the PIP joint immediately after surgery. Most surgical techniques require the DIP to be immobilized for 4 to 8 weeks, but the patient may return to work immediately provided that hard labor is not involved.[22]

SUMMARY

We prefer wide-awake finger fracture reduction, closed percutaneous K-wire fixation, and early protected movement to treat phalangeal fractures. This approach allows intraoperative visualization of active movement after K-wire fixation with the possibility of adjustments during the case. It also negates the need for extensive dissection with subsequent scar formation between the tendons and the bone. It provides the same advantages that are provided by early protected movement after flexor tendon repair.

SUPPLEMENTARY DATA

Supplementary data related to this article can be found online at http://dx.doi.org/32.1016/j.hcl.2013.08.014.

REFERENCES

1. Jones NF, Jupiter JB, Lalonde DH. Common fractures and dislocations of the hand. Plast Reconstr Surg 2012;130:722e–36e.
2. Chung KC, Spilson SV. The frequency and epidemiology of hand and forearm fractures in the United States. J Hand Surg Am 2001;26:908–15.
3. Belsky MR, Eaton RG, Lane LB. UBC-IT's Shibboleth Identity Provider v2.2. J Hand Surg 1984 Sep;9: 725–9.
4. Al-Qattan MM. Closed reduction and percutaneous K-wires versus open reduction and interosseous loop wires for displaced unstable transverse fractures of the shaft of the proximal phalanx of the fingers in industrial workers. J Hand Surg 2008;33: 552–6.

5. Faruqui S, Stern PJ, Kiefhaber TR. Percutaneous pinning of fractures in the proximal third of the proximal phalanx: complications and outcomes. J Hand Surg Am 2012;37:1342–8.
6. Al-Qattan MM. K-wire fixation for extraarticular transverse/short oblique fractures of the shaft of the middle phalanx associated with extensor tendon injury. J Hand Surg 2008;33:561–5.
7. Horton T. A prospective randomized controlled study of fixation of long oblique and spiral shaft fractures of the proximal phalanx: closed reduction and percutaneous Kirschner wiring versus open reduction and lag screw fixation. J Hand Surg 2003;28:5–9.
8. Suzuki Y, Matsunaga T, Sato S, et al. The pins and rubbers traction system for treatment of comminuted intraarticular fractures and fracture-dislocations in the hand. J Hand Surg Br 1994;19:98–107.
9. Ruland RT, Hogan CJ, Cannon DL, et al. Use of dynamic distraction external fixation for unstable fracture-dislocations of the proximal interphalangeal joint. J Hand Surg Am 2008;33(1):19–25. Available at: ScienceDirect.com.
10. Dionysian E, Eaton RG. The long-term outcome of volar plate arthroplasty of the proximal interphalangeal joint. J Hand Surg Am 2000;25:429–37.
11. Afendras G, Abramo A, Mrkonjic A, et al. Hemi-hamate osteochondral transplantation in proximal interphalangeal dorsal fracture dislocations: a minimum 4 year follow-up in eight patients. J Hand Surg Am 2010;35:627–31.
12. Wu WC, Fok MW, Fung KY, et al. Autologous osteochondral graft for traumatic defects of finger joints. J Hand Surg Am 2012;37:251–7.
13. Calfee RP, Kiefhaber TR, Sommerkamp TG. Hemi-hamate arthroplasty provides functional reconstruction of acute and chronic proximal interphalangeal fracture-dislocations. J Hand Surg Am 2009;34(7): 1232–41. Available at: ScienceDirect.com.
14. Newington D. The treatment of dorsal fracture-dislocation of the proximal interphalangeal joint by closed reduction and Kirschner wire fixation: a 16-year follow up. J Hand Surg 2001;26:537–40.
15. Inoue G, Tamura Y. Treatment of fracture-dislocation of the proximal interphalangeal joint using extension-block Kirschner wire. Ann Chir Main Memb Super 1991;10(6):564–8. Available at: ScienceDirect.com.
16. Edwards GS, O'Brien ET, Heckman MM. Retrograde cross-pinning of transverse metacarpal and phalangeal fractures. Hand 1982;14:141–8.
17. Paksima N, Johnson J, Brown A, et al. Percutaneous pinning of middle phalangeal neck fractures: surgical technique. J Hand Surg Am 2012;37:1913–6.
18. Hamas RS, Horrell ED, Pierret GP. Treatment of mallet finger due to intra-articular fracture of the distal phalanx. J Hand Surg Am 1978;3:361–3.
19. Ishiguro T, Imai N, Tomatsu T, et al. A new method of closed reduction using the spring action of Kirschner wires for fractures of the tibial plateau–a preliminary report. Nihon Seikeigeka Gakkai Zasshi 1986;60:227–36.
20. Pegoli L. The Ishiguro extension block technique for the treatment of mallet finger fracture: indications and clinical results. J Hand Surg 2003;28:15–7.
21. Darderprats A, Fernandezgarcia E, Fernandezgabarda R, et al. Treatment of mallet finger fractures by the extension-block K-wire technique. J Hand Surg 1998;23:802–5.
22. Lee SK, Kim KJ, Yang DS, et al. Modified extension-block K-wire fixation technique for the treatment of bony mallet finger. Orthopedics 2010;33(10):728.
23. Tetik C, Gudemez E. Modification of the extension block Kirschner wire technique for mallet fractures. Clin Orthop Relat Res 2002;284–90.
24. Badia A, Riano F. A simple fixation method for unstable bony mallet finger. J Hand Surg 2004;29:1051–5.
25. Rocchi L, Genitiempo M, Fanfani F. Percutaneous fixation of mallet fractures by the "umbrella handle" technique. J Hand Surg 2006;31:407–12.
26. Schneider LH. Fractures of the distal phalanx. Hand Clin 1988;4:537–47.
27. Gaston RG, Chadderdon C. Phalangeal fractures: displaced/nondisplaced. Hand Clin 2012;28(3):395–401.
28. Yeo CJ, Sebastin SJ, Chong AK. Fingertip injuries. Singapore Med J 2010;51:78–86 [quiz: 7].
29. Hornbach E. Closed reduction and percutaneous pinning of fractures of the proximal phalanx. J Hand Surg 2001;26:45–9.
30. Elmaraghy MW, Elmaraghy AW, Richards RS, et al. Transmetacarpal intramedullary K-wire fixation of proximal phalangeal fractures. Ann Plast Surg 1998;41:125.
31. Al-Qattan MM. Displaced unstable transverse fractures of the shaft of the proximal phalanx of the fingers in industrial workers: reduction and K-wire fixation leaving the metacarpophalangeal and proximal interphalangeal joints free. J Hand Surg 2011;36:577–83.
32. Pun WK, Chow SP, So YC, et al. Unstable phalangeal fractures: treatment by A.O. screw and plate fixation. J Hand Surg Am 1991;16(1):113–7. Available at: ScienceDirect.com.
33. Aladin A, Davis T. Dorsal fracture? Dislocation of the proximal interphalangeal joint: a comparative study of percutaneous Kirschner wire fixation versus open reduction and internal fixation. J Hand Surg 2005;30:120–8.
34. Ikeda M, Kobayashi Y, Mochida J, et al. Percutaneous pinning of the displaced volar plate avulsion fracture of the PIP joint. Hand Surg 2009;14:113–9.
35. Waris E, Alanen V. Percutaneous, intramedullary fracture reduction and extension block pinning for dorsal proximal interphalangeal fracture-dislocations. J Hand Surg Am 2010;35:2046–52.
36. Crawford GP. The molded polythene splint for mallet finger deformities. J Hand Surg Am 1984;9:231–7.

Minimally Invasive Treatment of Raynaud Phenomenon
The Role of Botulinum Type A

Michael W. Neumeister, MD, FRCSC*,
Kelli Nicole Belangee Webb, MD, Michael Romanelli, BS

KEYWORDS

• Minimally invasive • Botulinum type A • Raynaud phenomenon • Treatment

KEY POINTS

- Although the mechanism is unknown, botulinum toxin type A injection may be an effective, localized, nonsurgical treatment option without addictive properties or systemic side effects for the treatment of ischemic digits.
- Clinical research supports the safety and efficacy of injection of botulinum toxin type A for the treatment of Raynaud phenomenon.

RAYNAUD PHENOMENON

Approximately 3% of the US population (9.15 million people) is affected by Raynaud phenomenon.[1] This vasospastic disorder is 9 times more common in females and typically occurs between 15 and 40 years of age.[2,3] Patients with Raynaud have an exaggerated vasoconstriction of their digital arteries in response to certain environmental triggers, which leads to pale, cold, numb, and sometimes painful, ulcerated digits (**Fig. 1**). Vasospastic episodes may be triggered by emotion, stress, coldness, trauma, moisture, smoking, or mild changes in ambient temperature.[4] These episodic attacks can last minutes to hours and may reoccur several times throughout the day. For most patients, these symptoms are simply bothersome; but for 1 out of 5 patients, the symptoms are so severe that they seek medical attention, most commonly for severe ischemic pain or fingertip ulcerations. The resultant digit ischemia may be associated with considerable morbidity: pain, ulcerations, loss of function, disability, and depression.[5–10]

Raynaud phenomenon can be classified into primary and secondary conditions.[5] Primary Raynaud is an idiopathic condition with no known associated comorbidity. Secondary Raynaud, however, is associated with other autoimmune or connective tissue disorders, such as scleroderma, mixed connective tissue disease, lupus, or Sjögren syndrome.[11] The pathophysiology of Raynaud phenomenon is still poorly understood. Primary vascular dysfunction, however, has been implicated as the essential physiologic abnormality in Raynaud phenomenon characterized by an imbalance between vasodilation and vasoconstriction. The vasospastic episodes are hypothesized as being under both sympathetic neural and chemical imbalances.[5]

Avoidance of exacerbating factors, especially cold and stress, are paramount to the management of Raynaud. If the condition is secondary to autoimmune or connective tissue disorders, these conditions should be medically managed and optimized through the patients' rheumatologists. The pharmacologic treatment of the ischemic digits has included such options as calcium channel blockers, nitric oxide, angiotensin-converting enzyme inhibitors, selective-serotonin receptor inhibitors, alpha-adrenergic blockers, anticoagulants, oral prostanoids, antithrombotics, phosphodiesterase type 5 inhibitors, endoltheial-1 receptor

Department of Surgery - Institute for Plastic Surgery, SIU School of Medicine, 747 North Rutledge 3rd Floor, PO Box 19653, Springfield, IL 62794, USA
* Corresponding author.
E-mail address: mneumeister@siumed.edu

Hand Clin 30 (2014) 17–24
http://dx.doi.org/10.1016/j.hcl.2013.09.006
0749-0712/14/$ – see front matter

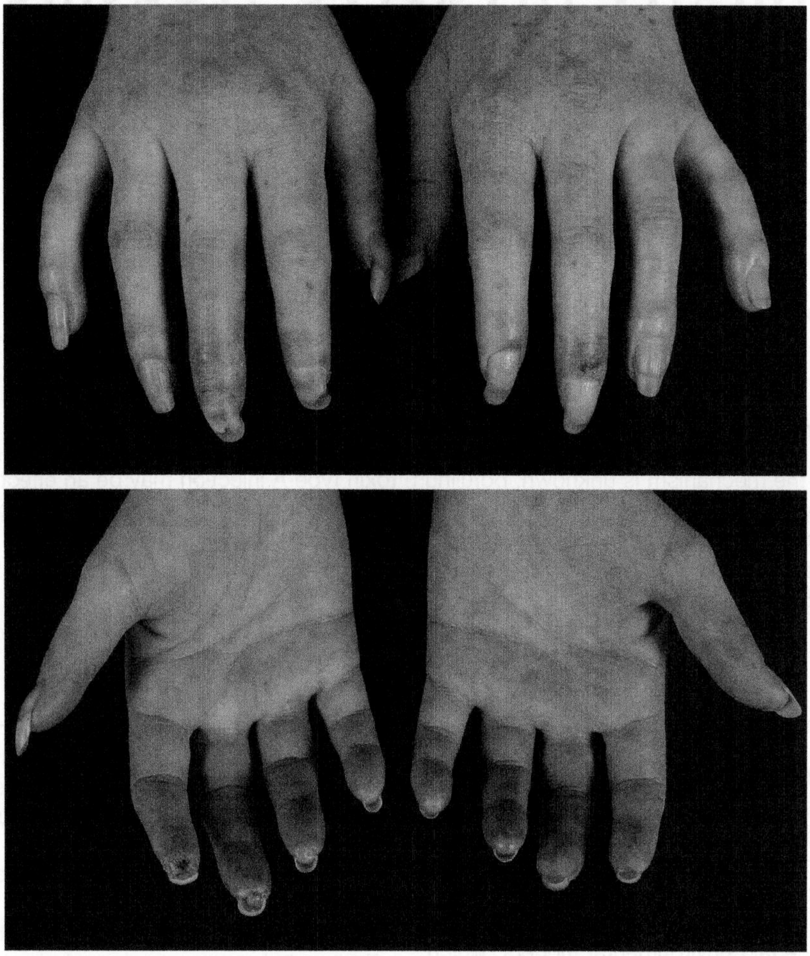

Fig. 1. Patients with Raynaud phenomenon are subject to extreme episodes of vasoconstriction of the digital arteries that results in discoloration, pain, stiffness, and ulcerations. (*From* Neumeister M. Botulinum toxin type A in the treatment of Raynaud's phenomenon. J Hand Surg 2010;35A:2086; with permission.)

antagonists, topical glyceryl trinitrate, and antioxidants.[5–7,11–18] Patients with severe pain and digit ulceration who have failed conservative managements are often referred to hand surgeons for further evaluation and treatment. Cervical sympathectomy was a surgical treatment option that has now fallen out of favor because of potential complications and poor long-term results.[4] Adrian Flatt[19] introduced digital sympathectomies for chronic ischemia whereby the vessels are surgically stripped of the adventitia and sympathetic innervation. The intent is to deny the digital artery of its potential to vasoconstrict. More aggressive peripheral artery and digital artery sympathectomies are more expansive and involve stripping the adventitia from the arteries at the level of the digital artery, palmar common digital artery, palmar arch, and/or radial and ulnar arteries. These sympathectomies, however, provide inconsistent or temporary relief and may be associated with surgical morbidity, such as contractures, stiffness, nerve injury, or vascular disruption.[7,19–21] Partial or full amputations may be necessary to relieve recalcitrant pain and ulcerations with exposed phalanges.

Over the last 10 years, many hand surgeons have demonstrated pain relief and ulcer healing with injection of botulinum toxin type A (Btx-A) around the neurovascular bundles of affected digits.[22] Btx-A injection is a much less invasive and less expensive option compared with surgical interventions, such as sympathectomies, and may provide immediate and long-term results.

INDICATIONS AND CONTRAINDICATIONS

The indications for the use of Btx-A in digital ischemia include Raynaud phenomenon and vascular insufficiencies not amenable to surgical bypass. The contraindications are listed in **Box 1**.

Box 1
The contraindications for the use of Btx-A in patients

- Known allergies
- Pregnancy
- Breast-feeding mothers
- Active infection
- Myasthenia gravis
- Patients on medications that decrease neuromuscular transmission
  - Calcium channel blockers
  - Penicillamine
  - Aminoglycosides
  - Licoamides
  - Polymyxins
  - Magnesium sulfate
  - Anticholinesterases
  - Succinylcholine
  - Quinidine

Although the US Food and Drug Administration has approved 8 different uses for Btx-A (**Table 1**), numerous off-label uses have been documented in the literature (**Box 2**). It should be clearly noted that Btx-A for the use in Raynaud phenomenon is also an off-label use of this medication.

METHOD OF TREATMENT

Btx-A is supplied in a small vial containing 50 to 100 units of the toxin. The contents of the vial must be reconstituted with preservative-free normal saline. Typically10 to 20 mL of the saline is used for the reconstitution so that there is roughly 5 to 10 units/mL. Using a 10-mL syringe per hand, about 2 mL are injected around each neurovascular bundle at the level of the metacarpophalangeal (MCP) joint. The idea is to bathe the neurovascular bundle with the 2 mL of Btx-A (**Fig. 2**). Only those digits that are symptomatic need to be injected. The Btx-A injection may produce temporary burning pain at the site of the injection. This pain typically lasts about 5 minutes. For this reason, wrist blocks with local anesthetic are commonly used today.

Complications of the injections may include temporary local pain, ecchymosis, or paralysis of the lumbrical and interosseous muscles. The paralysis of the intrinsic muscles is also temporary but may last for 2 to 3 months. Gross function is not impaired.

CLINICAL RESEARCH

Five retrospective case series, one case report, and numerous reviews have been published on the use of Btx-A in patients with Raynaud.[14,22–25] In 2004, Sycha and colleagues[25] reported the first pilot study of Btx-A injections into the hands of 2 patients with Raynaud phenomenon. In 2007, Van Beek and colleagues[16] published an article describing Btx-A injections in the hands of 11 patients with Raynaud phenomenon. They found that injecting Btx-A reduced patients' rest pain, promoted healing of digit ulcerations, and reduced the overall frequency of attacks that patients with Raynaud experienced.[7] In 2009, Fregene and colleagues[26] published an article describing Btx-A injections in the hands of 26 patients with Raynaud disease. They found that 75% of patients experienced a significant reduction in pain, 56%

Table 1
Summary of FDA-approved botulinum toxin products

Trade Name	NEW Drug Name	OLD Drug Name	Indication
Botox	OnabotulinumtoxinA	Botulinum toxin type A	Cervical dystonia Axillary hyperhidrosis Strabismus Blepharospasm Urinary incontinence Migraine headache Upper limb spasticity
Botox Cosmetic	OnabotulinumtoxinA	Botulinum toxin type A	Glabellar rhytids
Dysport	OnabotulinumtoxinA	Botulinum toxin type A	Cervical dystonia Glabellar rhytids
Myobloc	RimabotulinumtoxinB	Botulinum toxin type B	Cervical dystonia

Box 2
Off-label uses for botulinum toxin products

Achalasia
Anismus
Back pain
Carpal tunnel syndrome
Cerebral palsy–related limb spasticity
Chronic anal fissure
Chronic pain
Delayed gastric emptying
Dystonia
Enlarged prostate
Epilepsy
Epiphora
Essential tremor
Fibromyalgia
Hereditary paraplegia
Interstitial cystitis
Ischemic digits
Lateral epicondylitis
Piriformis syndrome
Pruritus
Raynaud phenomenon
Rhinitis
Sialorrhea
Spasmodic dysphonia
Stuttering
Tardive dyskinesia
Tourette syndrome
Vaginismus

experienced improvement in transcutaneous oxygen saturation, 48% of ulcers healed within 9.5 weeks, and 89% of patients experienced improvements after 1 treatment. In July 2009, Neumeister and colleagues[27] published the effects of Btx-A in 19 patients. Sixteen of 19 patients reported resolution of pain, all chronic ulcers healed within 60 days of injection, and 84% noticed an immediate increase in finger perfusion. In 2010, Neumeister reported pain relief and increased perfusion of digits in 28 of 33 patients treated with Btx-A for Raynaud phenomenon (**Figs. 3** and **4**, **Table 2**).[28]

Each study reported that most (75%–100%) of the patients had pain relief following the Btx-A

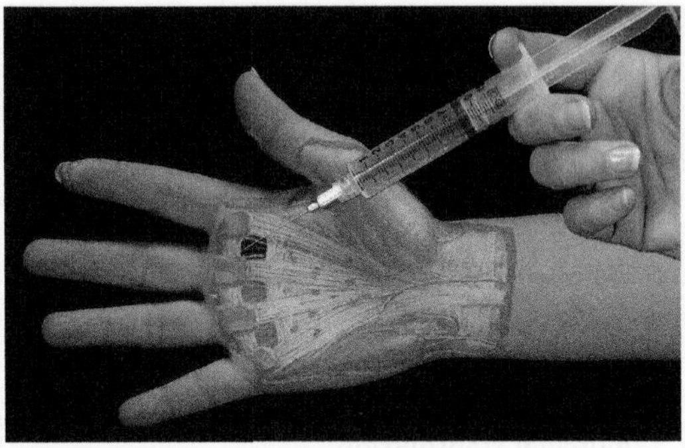

Fig. 2. Preservative-free normal saline is used to reconstitute the Btx-A. This schematic demonstrates 10 mL of saline mixed with the 100 units of Btx-A; 2 mL are injected around each neurovascular bundle at the level of the bifurcation of the common digital vessels around the MCP joint. (*From* Neumeister M. Botulinum toxin type A in the treatment of Raynaud's phenomenon. J Hand Surg 2010;35A:2087; with permission.)

injections. The onset of pain relief was reported within minutes to 48 hours. The duration of pain relief was variable from months to more than 6 years without recurrence. A few patients required repeat injections for recurrence of the painful episodes. All responding patients had fewer and less severe episodes than before the Btx-A injections. Ischemic ulcers healed in 48% to 100% of patients.

The authors are currently conducting a prospective, randomized, double-blind, placebo-controlled trial on Btx-A for treatment of Raynaud phenomenon. The results of this study will likely refine and expand the indications for the use of Btx-A to treat these patients.

BASIC SCIENCE RESEARCH

Btx-A is a protein and neurotoxin derived from the bacterium Clostridium botulinum that paralyzes muscle.[25,29] Btx-A blocks the release of acetylcholine across nerve terminals to the motor muscle units (**Fig. 5**).[6] This process typically has a delay of 1 to 4 days, which is the reason paralysis is not clinically evident for that duration of time. Btx-A is taken up by the synaptic nerve terminal by endocytosis and eventually binds to a fusion protein called synaptosomal associated protein–25 (SNAP-25) located on the acetylcholine vesicle. These fusion proteins permit the docking of the vesicles to the end on the nerve terminal to commence exocytosis of the neurotransmitter. The SNAP-25 is proteolytically degraded by Btx-A, which immobilizes the vesicle so it is unable to anchor to the nerve membrane and release the acetylcholine across the

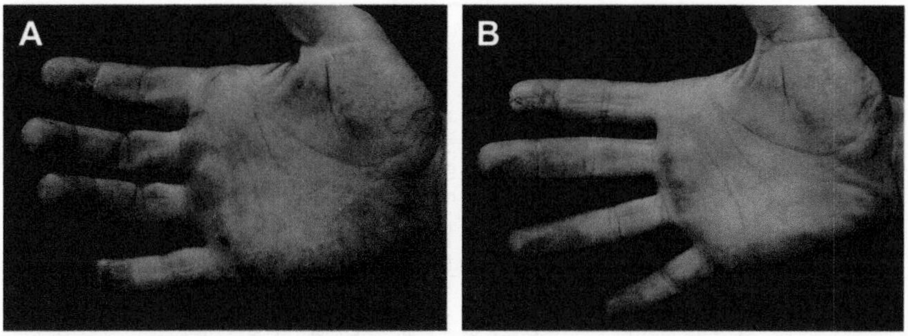

Fig. 3. (*A, B*). Preinjection (*A*) and postinjection (*B*) of Btx-A for ischemic digits. Perfusion is enhanced with a corresponding systemic relief of pain. (*From* Neumeister M, Chambers C, Herron M, et al. Botox therapy for ischemic digits. Plast Reconstr Surg 2009;124(1):194; with permission.)

neuromuscular junction. This effect lasts 2 to 4 months until new SNAP-25 proteins on the vesicles are formed.

Btx-A injection for the treatment of patients with ischemia and pain seen in Raynaud disease, however, has almost immediate and extremely prolonged effects. This fact must mean that, in Raynaud disease, Btx-A is working by a different mechanism. The effects of Btx-A in Raynaud may be related to antinociceptive effects on nerves directly or their neurotransmitters. It has been postulated that Btx-A may affect several pain-related neurotransmitters, including norepinephrine, substance P, glutamate, and calcitonin gene-related protein (CGRP).[15,30–32] Btx-A has P, +glutamate, and +CGRP, all known pain transmission peptides that communicate with the spinal cord and the cerebral cortex.[15,30] This point may mean the effects of Btx-A injections are related to the local or central blockade of neurotransmitters upregulated in states of chronic nerve irritation and pain. Additionally, the effects of Btx-A on the improved vascularity of the ischemic digits may be sympathetically mediated. If Btx-A blocks substance P, it may decrease or abolish the self-perpetuating cycle of pain and sympathetic stimulation. Finally, there may also be direct or indirect crosstalk between the A and C fibers in the dorsal root ganglion, a method of communication known as *ephapses*.[12,15,33] In fact, numerous chemical and anatomic changes have been observed within the dorsal root ganglion in chronic pain models.[34] It is conceivable that Btx-A has more than one mode of pain inhibition and may be acting at several sites. By the blockade of neurotransmitters, or ectopic Na+ channels on chronically irritated nerves, or through its effect on microvascularity, Btx-A has a distinct role in pain reduction in patients with Raynaud.[15]

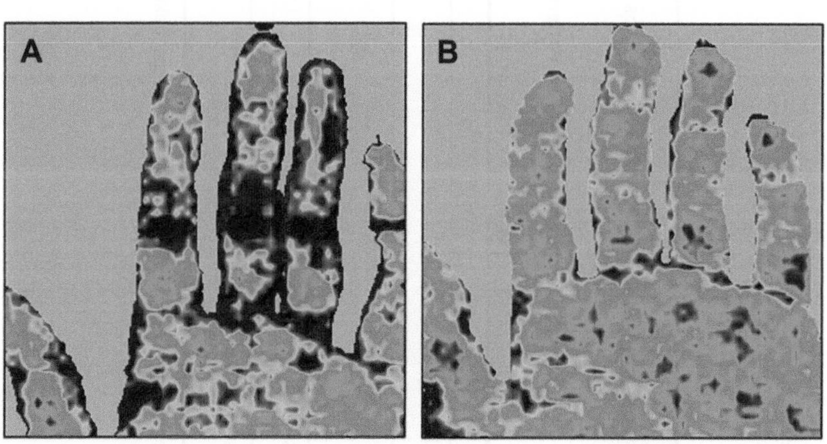

Fig. 4. (*A, B*). A laser Doppler scan to quantify the changes in perfusion following Btx-A injection. Preinjection (*A*) and postinjection (*B*) of the Btx-A. The red and yellow color demonstrates greater perfusion after the injection. (*From* Neumeister M. Botulinum toxin type A in the treatment of Raynaud's phenomenon. J Hand Surg 2010;35A:2088; with permission.)

Table 2
Summary of findings from 4 retrospective studies using injected Btx-A to Raynaud phenomenon

Study	No. of Patients (M/F)	No. of Patients with 1°/2° Raynaud	Avg Age in Years (Range)	Percent with Symptomatic Relief (No.)	Length of Follow-up in Months: Avg (Max)	Avg Duration Pain Relief in Months (Range)	Complications No. (%)
Sycha et al,[23] 2004	2 (0/2)	1/1	50.5 (19–63)	100 (2/2)	1.75 (2)	1.75 (1.5–2.0)	None
Van Beek et al,[16] 2007	11 (2/9)	1/10	50.8 (23–70)	100 (11/11)	9.6 (30)	Not reported	Temporary intrinsic muscle weakness: 3 (27%)
Fregene et al,[26] 2009	26 (12/14)	15/11	55.0 (37–72)	75 (19/6)	18 (45)	Not reported	Temporary intrinsic muscle weakness: 6 (23%) Transient dysesthesia: 1 (4%)
Neumeister et al,[27] 2009	19 (7/12)	13/6	44.1 (15–72)	84 (16/19)	Not Reported (59)	23.4 (0.5–59.0)	Temporary intrinsic muscle weakness: 3 (16%)
Neumeister et al,[28] 2010	33 (14,19)	23/10	43.0 (15–72)	84 (28/33)	(103)	(0.5–103.0)	Temporary intrinsic muscle weakness: 7 (21%)

Abbreviations: Avg, average; F, female; M, male; Max, maximum.

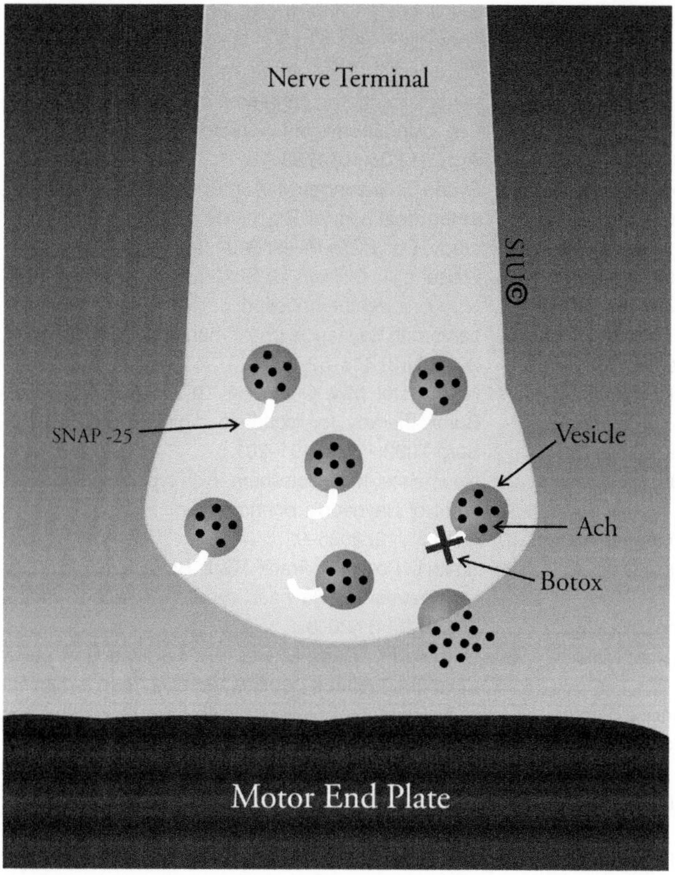

Fig. 5. The classic mechanism of action of Btx-A that promotes muscle paralysis. Btx-A is taken up by the nerve terminal and prevents the release of acetylcholine needed to stimulate muscle contracture. Btx-A binds to a fusion protein called *synaptosomal associated protein-25* (SNAP-25) located on the acetylcholine neurotransmitter vesicle. The vesicle is rendered incapable of migrating to the end of the nerve terminal and releasing the acetylcholine. (*From* Neumeister M. Botulinum toxin type A in the treatment of Raynaud's phenomenon. J Hand Surg 2010;35A:2091, with permission; and Neumeister M, Chambers C, Herron M, et al. Botox therapy for ischemic digits. Plast Reconstr Surg 2009;124(1):198, with permission.)

SUMMARY

Although the mechanism is unknown, Btx-A injection may be an effective, localized, nonsurgical treatment option without addictive properties or systemic side effects for the treatment of ischemic digits. Clinical research supports the safety and efficacy of injection of Btx-A for the treatment of Raynaud phenomenon.

REFERENCES

1. Department of Health and Human Services, Public Health Service, National Institutes of Health, et al. Questions and answers about Raynaud's phenomenon. NIH Publication No. 06–4911. 2001; Revised June 2006. Available at: http://www.niams.nih.gov/Health Info/Raynauds Phenomenon.
2. Coffman JD. Raynaud's phenomenon. Curr Treat Options Cardiovasc Med 2000;2(3):219–26.
3. de Trafford JC, Lafferty K, Potter CE, et al. An epidemiological survey of Raynaud's phenomenon. Eur J Vasc Surg 1988;2:167–70.
4. Coveliers HM, Hoexum F, Nederhoed JH, et al. Thoracic sympathectomy for digital ischemia: a summary of evidence. J Vasc Surg 2011;54(1):273–7.
5. Herrick AL. Pathogenesis of Raynaud's phenomenon. Rheumatology 2005;44:587–96.
6. Herrick AL. Management of Raynaud's phenomenon and digital ischemia. Curr Rheumatol Rep 2013;15(1):303.
7. Koman LA, Smith BP, Smith TL. Vascular disorders. In: Green DP, Hotchkiss RN, Pederson WC, editors. Greens operative hand surgery. New York: Churchill Livingstone; 1999. p. 2254–302.
8. O'Brien BM, Kumar PA, Mellow CG, et al. Radical microarteriolysis in the treatment of vasospastic disorders of the hand, especially scleroderma. J Hand Surg Br 1992;17(4):447–52.
9. Plante GE. Depression and cardiovascular disease: a reciprocal relationship. Metabolism 2005;54(5 Suppl 1):45–8.
10. Setler P. Therapeutic use of botulinum toxins: background and history. Clin J Pain 2002;18(6):S119–24.
11. Henness S, Wigley FM. Current drug therapy for scleroderma and secondary Raynaud's

phenomenon: evidence-based review. Curr Opin Rheumatol 2007;19(6):611–8.
12. Alfredson H, Lorentzon R. Chronic tendon pain: no signs of chemical inflammation but high concentrations of the neurotransmitter glutamate. Implications for treatment? Curr Drug Targets 2002;3(1):43–54.
13. Bergstrom KG, Perelman RO. Treatment for Raynaud's: beyond calcium channel blockers. J Drugs Dermatol 2008;7(5):497–500.
14. Levien TL. Advances in the treatment of Raynaud's phenomenon. Vasc Health Risk Manag 2010;6: 167–77.
15. McMahon HT, Foran P, Dolly JO, et al. Tetanus toxin and botulinum toxins type A and B inhibit glutamate, gamma-aminobutyric acid, aspartate, and met-enkephalin release from synaptosomes. Clues to the locus of action. J Biol Chem 1992;267(30): 21338–43.
16. Van Beek AL, Lim PK, Gear AJ, et al. Management of vasospastic disorders with botulinum toxin A. Plast Reconstr Surg 2007;119:217.
17. Thompson AE, Pope JE. Calcium channel blockers for primary Raynaud's phenomenon: a meta-analysis. Rheumatology 2005;44:145–50.
18. Wall LB, Stern P. Nonoperative treatment of digital ischemia in systemic sclerosis. J Hand Surg Am 2012;37(9):1907–9.
19. Flatt AE. Digital artery sympathectomy. J Hand Surg Am 1980;5(6):550–6.
20. Dorafshar AH, Seitz IA, Zachary L. Reoperative digital sympathectomy in refractory Raynaud's phenomenon. Plast Reconstr Surg 2009;123(1): 36e–8e.
21. Hartzell TL, Makhni EC, Sampson C. Long-term results of peripheral sympathectomy. J Hand Surg Am 2009;34(8):1454–60.
22. Iorio ML, Masden DL, Higgins JP. Botulinum toxin A treatment of Raynaud's phenomenon: a review. Semin Arthritis Rheum 2012;41(4):599–603.
23. Kossintseva I, Barankin B. Improvement in both Raynaud disease and hyperhidrosis in response to botulinum toxin A treatment. J Cutan Med Surg 2008;12(4):189–93.
24. Mannava S, Plate JF, Stone AV, et al. Recent advances for the management of Raynaud phenomenon using botulinum neurotoxin A. J Hand Surg Am 2011;36(10):1708–10.
25. Sycha T, Graninger M, Auff E, et al. Botulinum toxin in the treatment of Raynaud's phenomenon: a pilot study. Eur J Clin Invest 2004;34:312–3.
26. Fregene A, Ditmars D, Siddiqui A. Botulinum toxin type A: a treatment option for digital ischemia in patients with Raynaud's phenomenon. J Hand Surg Am 2009;34(3):446–52.
27. Neumeister MW, Chambers CB, Herron MS, et al. Botox therapy for ischemic digits. Plast Reconstr Surg 2009;124(1):191–201.
28. Neumeister MW. Botulinum toxin type A in the treatment of Raynaud's phenomenon. J Hand Surg Am 2010;35(12):2085–92.
29. Smith L, Polsky D, Frank AG Jr. Botulinum toxin-A for the treatment of Raynaud syndrome. Arch Dermatol 2012;148(4):426–8.
30. Durham PL, Cady R, Cady R. Regulation of calcitonin gene-related peptide secretion from trigeminal nerve cells by botulinum toxin type A: implications for migraine therapy. Headache 2004;44(1):35–42 [discussion: 42–3].
31. Edwards CM, Marshall JM, Pugh M. Cardiovascular responses evoked mild cool stimuli in primary Raynaud's disease: the role of endothelin. Clin Sci 1999;96:577.
32. Leppert J, Ringqvist A, Ahlner J. Seasonal variations in cyclic GMP response on whole-body cooling in women with primary Raynaud's phenomenon. Clin Sci 1997;93:175.
33. Cui M, Khanijou S, Rubino J, et al. Subcutaneous administration of botulinum toxin A reduces formalin-induced pain. Pain 2004;107:125–33.
34. Devor M, Wall PD. Cross-excitation in dorsal root ganglia of nerve-injured and intact rats. J Neurophysiol 1990;64(6):1733–46.

Collagenase Injections for Treatment of Dupuytren Disease

Vincent R. Hentz, MD

KEYWORDS

• Dupuytren • Contracture • Collagenase • Injection

KEY POINTS

- Food and Drug Administration (FDA) and manufacturer inclusion criteria include a palpable cord causing at least a 20° contracture of a metacarpophalangeal (MP) or proximal interphalangeal (PIP) joint.
- Pay strict attention to the injection technique. Strive to inject only into the cord.
- Inform patients regarding the inevitable onset of side effects—pain, swelling, and bruising—and their expected duration.
- Use local anesthesia for manipulation.
- Long-standing PIP joint contractures benefit from postinjection directed hand therapy and dynamic splinting.

INTRODUCTION: NATURE OF THE PROBLEM

Dupuytren disease (DD) is a benign, generally painless connective tissue disorder affecting the palmar fascia that leads to progressive hand contractures. Mediated by myofibroblasts, the disease most commonly begins as a nodule in the palm or finger. If the disease progresses, pathologic cords form leading to progressive flexion deformity of the involved fingers, commonly of the MP and PIP joints but also of the distal interphalangeal (DIP) joint and the first web space. The palmar skin overlying the cords may become excessively calloused and contracted and involved joints may develop periarticular fibrosis. This is particularly true of the PIP joints. Although there is as yet no cure, the sequellae of this affliction can be corrected.

Treatment of DD was first described by Henry Cline[1] in the late seventeenth century and involved sectioning the pathologic cords, later known as fasciotomy or aponeurotomy. Since then, surgical intervention traditionally has been the most effective and widely accepted treatment of progressive contracture. Today's surgical options include limited percutaneous needle aponeurectomy (NA), open versus percutaneous fasciotomy, and the more commonly performed open fasciectomy. Collagenase clostridium histolyticum (CCH) was introduced to the literature slightly more than 15 years ago[2] as a potential minimally invasive, nonsurgical option to treat Dupuytren contractures (DCs). This has ultimately led to completion of phase III clinical trials and its recent US FDA approval for clinical use under the marketed name, Xiaflex; in Europe, the drug is marketed as Xiapex. The remainder of this article focuses on the author's experience and recommendations with collagenase fasciotomy as a minimally invasive technology to treat DCs of the MP and PIP joints.

The author has nothing to disclose.
Robert A. Chase Center for Hand and Upper Limb Surgery, Stanford University, 770 Welch Road, Suite 400, Palo Alto, CA 94304, USA
E-mail address: vrhentz@stanford.edu

Hand Clin 30 (2014) 25–32
http://dx.doi.org/10.1016/j.hcl.2013.08.016
0749-0712/14/$ – see front matter

INDICATIONS/CONTRAINDICATIONS

Indications

FDA and manufacturer treatment guidelines include the presence of a palpable cord causing at least a 20° contracture of an MP or PIP joint.

Contraindications

- The procedure is not painless and patients intolerant of pain are poor candidates.
- The drug is expensive. Only one cord is treated at a time. Patients with multiple cords potentially face months of treatment and considerable expense.
- No history or evidence of sensitivity to the drug.

SURGICAL TECHNIQUE/PREPARING FOR INJECTION

Overview

Only a single dose can be administered at any one time and the dose must be injected directly into the specific (targeted) cord. The patient returns the following day or days to allow time for the collagenase to digest and lyse the collagen within the cord. An extension force is then applied to the involved finger to rupture the already weakened cord. FDA and manufacturer guidelines state that no more than 3 injections given at no less than monthly intervals may be used to affect improvement for the targeted joint.

Dosage and Injection Guidelines

CCH is supplied as a lyophilized powder with each vial containing 0.9 mg of CCH. Just prior to injection, the drug is reconstituted with sterile diluent consisting of 0.3 mg/mL of calcium chloride dihydrate and 0.9% sodium chloride. For MP joint contractures, a volume of 0.39 mL of sterile diluent is used for reconstitution and 0.58 mg of CCH in a total volume of 0.25 mL is injected into the targeted cord. For PIP joint contractures, 0.31 mL of sterile diluent is used for reconstitution and 0.58 mg of CCH in a total volume of 0.20 mL is injected into the targeted cord. Once reconstituted, CCH may be stored at room temperature for 1 hour or refrigerated for up to 4 hours.

PROCEDURE

Step One

Inject with a 1-mL syringe and a 0.5-in, 27-gauge needle. Local anesthesia is not recommended at the time of injection due to distortion of the soft tissue anatomy and the potential for deactivation of the drug.

Step Two

Use the nondominant hand to apply gentle extension to the finger undergoing injection, displacing the cord superficially away from the underlying flexor tendon mechanism.

Step Three

Insert the needle perpendicularly through the skin into the underlying cord. The tissue should be firm and resist easy passage of the needle.

Step Four

Passive manipulation of the PIP or DIP joint ensures that the needle has not been improperly positioned within the underlying flexor tendon. Inject one-third of the volume. Resistance to fluid flow indicates that the needle is within the cord.

Step Five

Withdraw the needle slightly, incline it distally, and reinsert into the cord approximately 3 mm from the site of the first aliquot. Confirm proper positioning and inject one-third of the dose.

Step Six

Reposition the needle 2 mm to 3 mm proximal to the initial injection and administer the final one-third of the dose (**Fig. 1**).

Pearls

The pretendinous cord causing an MP contracture should be injected where the cord is displaced the farthest from the MP joint and underlying flexor sheath (**Fig. 2**). This is typically midway between the distal palmar and palmodigital creases. Avoid injecting at the site of callosities because the skin is likely to tear on manipulation.

Inject cords causing PIP contractures just distal to the palmodigital crease. Avoid injecting more than 4 mm distal to the crease because injection more distal increases the risk of intratendinous injection.

IMMEDIATE POSTOPERATIVE CARE

I wrap the hand in a soft dressing as a reminder that patients should avoid hand-intensive activity for the next hours. Patients may resume a normal schedule that evening. I again categorize the likely side effects to preempt unnecessary postinjection patient concerns and late-night phone calls to me.

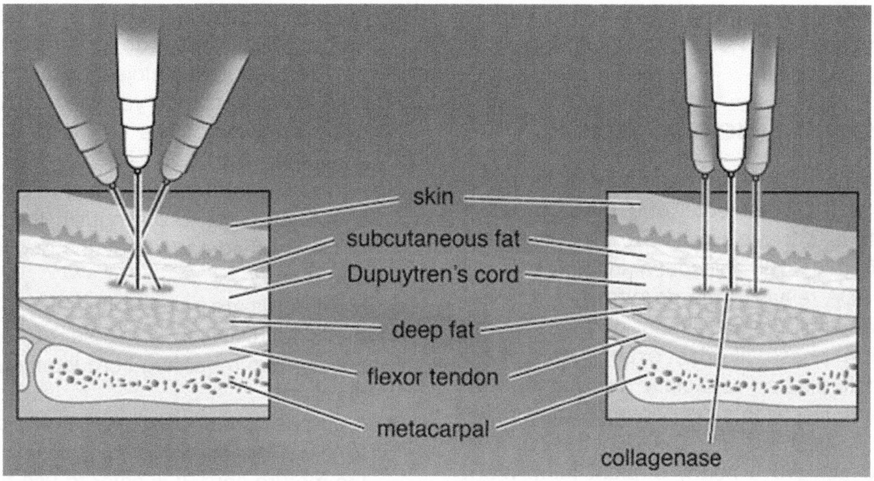

Fig. 1. Two different injection techniques are illustrated. The goal is to inject the total volume into the cord over a distance of 5–6 mm. (*From* Hentz VR, Watt AJ, Desai SS, et al. Advances in the management of Dupuytren disease: collagenase. Hand Clin 2012;28(4):552; with permission.)

I do not prescribe pain medication but rather recommend the use of acetaminophen or similar safe analgesics as necessary. Many patients assume that they will have full use of their hand the next day and must be cautioned that this is far from the case for most.

MANIPULATION

The manufacturer advises performing manipulation 24 hours after injection. I have varied the interval between injection and manipulation from 1 day to 1 week without seemingly altering the rate of success (**Table 1**). I use primarily intermetacarpal blockade with 1% xylocaine at the time of manipulation to facilitate patient comfort. I manipulate MP joint contractures by applying firm passive extension, holding the finger in maximal extension for 10 to 20 seconds. Up to 3 attempts may be performed. For isolated PIP contractures, I first flex the MP joint prior to applying firm, passive extension across the PIP joint. If notable improvement occurs, patients are fitted with a nighttime extension splint to be worn for 4 weeks and instructed in passive extension exercises. No splint is worn

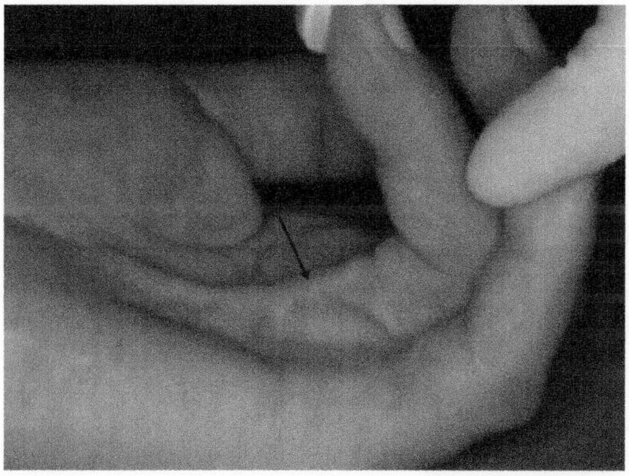

Fig. 2. A good candidate has an easily palpable pretendinous cord. The optimum site for injection is indicated by the arrow. (*From* Hentz VR, Watt AJ, Desai SS, et al. Advances in the management of Dupuytren disease: collagenase. Hand Clin 2012;28(4):554; with permission.)

Table 1
Comparison of joints manipulated at 24 hours postinjection versus those manipulated at 7 days postinjection

	Manipulation at 1 d (N = 25)	Manipulation at 7 d (N = 25)
Number of MPJs	14	13
Pre-Rx angle	47°	46°
Post-Rx angle	11°	9°
Number of PIPJs	11	12
Pre-Rx angle	56°	53°
Post-Rx angle	25°	16°
Spontaneous ruptures		
MPJs	7%	58%
PIPJs	0%	33%
Number of skin tears	0	3

Abbreviations: MPJ, MP joint; PIPJ, PIP joint; Rx, treatment.
Spontaneous ruptures represent cords that ruptured without manipulation by the physician.

during the day and patients often return to active use of the hand within 3 to 5 days depending on comfort.

AUTHOR'S EXPERIENCE AND TECHNICAL TIPS

We were fortunate to be involved in both the 1999–2000 phase II (34 subjects) and the 2007–2008 phase III trials (39 subjects, >100 injections) and have performed 160 injections in 101 patients since the FDA released the drug for general use. Our clinical results mirror almost perfectly the results of the phase III trial, except for several notable differences, especially concerning PIP contractures. Recall that the phase III study called for up to 3 injections into the target cord in an attempt to achieve a nearly straight joint. Many study patients with PIP contractures had multiple injections. As we have gained experience, we have learned that most patients with either MP or PIP joint contractures are satisfied with almost any notable improvement and rarely ask to have a second injection. Our indications have both broadened and narrowed (discussed later).[3,4] This discussion is based on this still growing experience.

General Rules

1. You must have one clearly palpable cord as the target for injection and some degree of fixed joint contracture, meaning that you cannot fully passively extend the joint. Even if a patient cannot fully actively extend, if you can passively fully extend the joint, the cord may not respond to injection because at the time of manipulation you may not be able to exert sufficient force to rupture the now-weakened cord.
2. Although the needle is small and sharp, you should be able to distinguish the resistance to flow of fluid caused by the dense collagen of the cord.
3. Most cords are no more than 3–4 mm deep to the skin. Develop a sense of topographic anticipation regarding cord location and needle depth.
4. A surprising amount of force may be needed to inject the fluid into the dense collagen of the mature cord. It is safer to use both hands during the actual injection (**Fig. 3**). I prefer to passively extend the finger with the ulnar side of one hand. I control the syringe with the thumb and index finger of this hand help maintain the exact depth of the needle while the second hand pushes the plunger of the syringe. This reduces the risk of the needle advancing deeper into the tissues as the plunger is depressed and resistance to the flow of fluid is encountered. This also reduces the risk of suddenly encountering no resistance to fluid flow and inadvertently injecting the entire volume in one place.
5. Often it is easier and safer to make 3 separate skin punctures, 2–3 mm apart, rather than

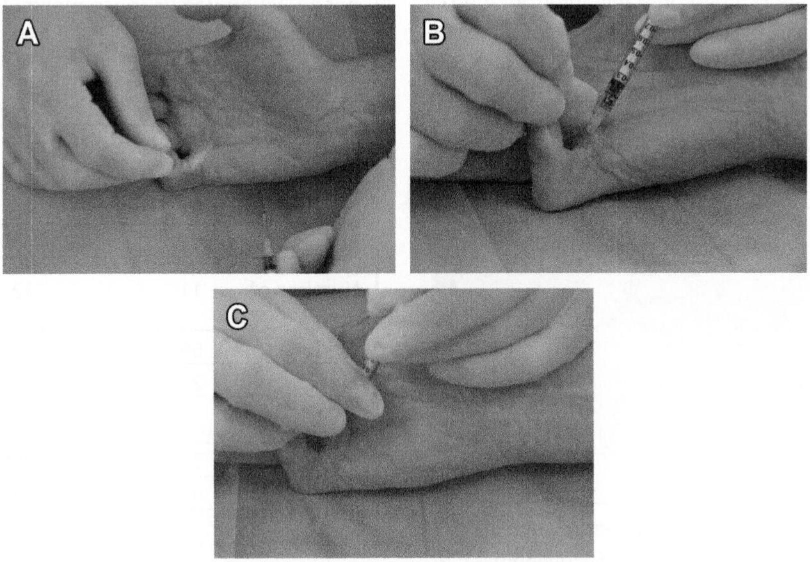

Fig. 3. The preferred 2-handed injection technique is illustrated. See text for description. The cord is delineated by palpation (*A*), the needle is inserted into the cord while tension is applied to the cord (*B*), and both hands support the syringe while the plunger is pressed (*C*). (*From* Hentz VR, Watt AJ, Desai SS, et al. Advances in the management of Dupuytren disease: collagenase. Hand Clin 2012;28(4):555; with permission.)

inclining the needle as the manufacturer's guidelines suggest.

6. Give patients some take-home information regarding the common side effects, such as pain, swelling, and bruising, and the less-common side effects, such as axillary lymphangitis. Reproduce some photographs of postinjection hands so that patients are fully informed. Advise mild analgesics at bedtime (**Fig. 4**).
7. The period between injection and manipulation can be varied considerably without negatively influencing the outcome (see **Table 1**). The cord remains weak for a yet-to-be-defined period of time postinjection.
8. When a patient comes for manipulation, examine the hand before injecting local anesthesia. The cord may have spontaneously ruptured.
9. We have operated on 4 former study patients who either had an inadequate response to injection or a recurrence. At surgery performed at least 1 year after injection, normal tissue planes were observed. It did not seem as if the injection had caused any residual scarring or alteration in the expected anatomy.
10. Review the billing and coding recommendations from the manufacturer or those suggested by the American Society for Surgery of the Hand. These are now 2 specific Current Procedural Terminology-4 codes created for this treatment. Obtain insurance preauthorization for patients who have private insurance. Be prepared for patient sticker shock from the US manufacturer's current charge for 1 vial (ie, 1 injection is $3200).

MP Joint Contractures

1. MP joint contractures almost always respond adequately to one injection. Rarely is a second injection needed, unless the first injection misses the cord. If the cord ruptures (or stretches notably) and the contracture corrects to a level of 60%–75% (usually <15° of residual contracture), no patient has asked for a second injection to correct the remaining few degrees of residual contraction. Patients are happy with this outcome. It is unwise to talk them into a second injection. Typically, not much more extension is gained unless they have a joint contracted both by its pretendinous cord and by a natatory cord arising from an adjacent digit's contracted pretendinous cord. In this case, the Y-shaped cord first should have been injected (as described).
2. If a Y-shaped cord is present and 2 adjacent digits are involved, inject at the confluence of the Y. You may achieve 2 corrected digits for the price and effort of a single injection (**Fig. 5**).
3. A tight natatory cord can be treated successfully. These can be more bothersome than

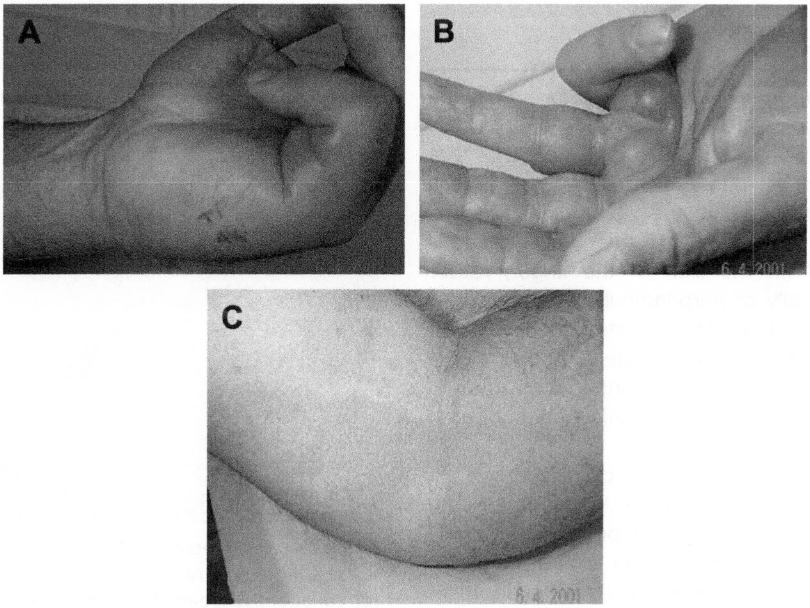

Fig. 4. (*A, B*) Demonstrate the hand 24 hours after injection. Note the edema and erythema. (*C*) Demonstrates the lymphangitis that some patients may experience. (*From* Hentz VR, Watt AJ, Desai SS, et al. Advances in the management of Dupuytren disease: collagenase. Hand Clin 2012;28(4):555; with permission.)

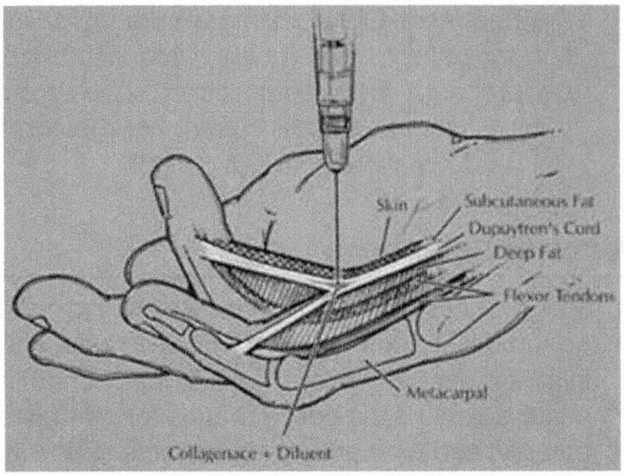

Fig. 5. The ideal site for injection when a Y-shaped cord is causing contracture of 2 adjacent digits is at the confluence of the Y. (*From* Hentz VR, Watt AJ, Desai SS, et al. Advances in the management of Dupuytren disease: collagenase. Hand Clin 2012;28(4): 560; with permission.)

pretendinous cords to piano players. Although technically off-label, natatory cords do not require 0.58 mg of drug. Look for another, possibly narrow, cord causing a contracture and consider splitting the dose.

4. The skin often tears with MP joint contractures greater than 50°, particularly if the skin overlying the cord is calloused. Prepare patients (and yourself) for this eventuality. All such tears have healed with simple wound care within 7–10 days. We have experienced far fewer skin tears when the interval between injection and manipulation is extended to 7 days.

PIP Contractures

1. All tendon ruptures experienced in the clinical trials occurred after multiple injections for fifth finger PIP contractures, usually for a central cords.[5] For a central cord, do not inject more than 4 mm distal to the palmodigital crease and consider inserting the needle more horizontally (from the side of the finger) rather than vertically or perpendicular to the palmar plane. Patients must understand this risk and practitioners must appreciate the implications of tendon rupture and reconstruction prior to incorporating collagenase injection into their practice.
2. The abductor digiti minimi cord is the most frequent cause of fifth finger PIP contractures. It is easily palpable and a good target for injection. It is always wide in the palmar to dorsal direction and you need to vary the depth of the 3 aliquots in this plane. The cord is well away from the flexor sheath and can be injected safely.
3. Lateral digital cords present good targets. Occasionally, radial and ulnar lateral digital cords coexist and cause PIP joint contracture. Weaken one and the other remains to maintain the joint contracted and resistant to manipulation. Consider splitting the dose and injecting both cords. This is also technically off-label.
4. Periarticular fibrosis is unaffected by collagenase. If the offending cord ruptures or softens and is no longer palpable, however, try dynamic splinting postinjection.
5. The PIP joint contracture associated with a huge nodule that practically fills the proximal phalanx does not respond to collagenase. I explain to patients that injecting a tiny volume of drug is akin to pouring a teacup of boiling water on the top of a glacier. A little ice melts but the glacier remains.
6. The recurrent PIP contracture associated with shrunken, scarred skin over the proximal phalanx is a poor candidate for collagenase (**Fig. 6**).
7. The extensor mechanism over the PIP joint becomes elongated in contractures that achieve 60°. The contracted PIP joint may, after injection and manipulation, be nearly fully passively correctable but patients will be unable to actively fully extend the joint and the contracture will recur to some degree quickly. Prolonged dynamic splinting may be helpful in achieving a more durable correction.[6]

Distal Interphalangeal Joint Contractures

I have had limited experience and have used a smaller dose of drug, with some success.

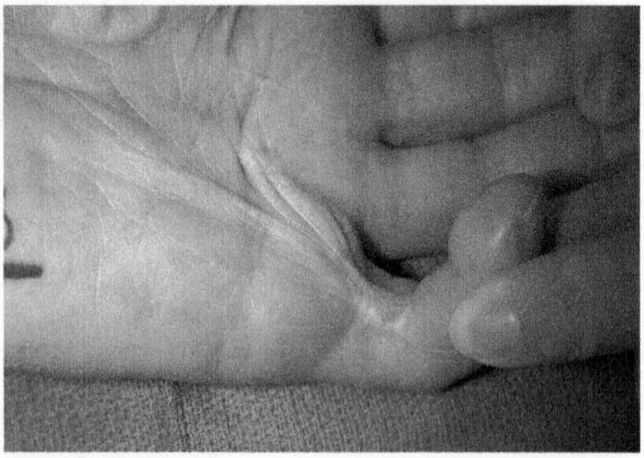

Fig. 6. A severe recurrent PIP contracture with badly scarred and contracted skin is a poor candidate for collagenase treatment. (*From* Hentz VR, Watt AJ, Desai SS, et al. Advances in the management of Dupuytren disease: collagenase. Hand Clin 2012;28(4):551–63; with permission.)

First Web-space Contractures

I have had mixed success in treating distal or proximal commissural cords. It seems difficult to exert enough tension on the cord at the time of manipulation.[7]

CLINICAL RESULTS IN THE LITERATURE

All results from both published and unpublished phases I, II, and III trials were combined in Auxilium's FDA report.[8] In total, 2630 collagenase injections were performed on 1780 cords in 1082 patients In all studies, MP joints responded significantly better than PIP joints. Later reports mirrored the results reported from the clinical trials. Witthaut and colleagues[9] reported the combined results from 2 open-label clinical trials with 879 treated joints treated with an average of 1.2 injections per affected joint. For MP joint contractures, 70% reached full or near-full extension compared with 37% of contracted PIP joints. Clinical improvement, defined as at least 50% correction, was achieved in 89% of MP contractures compared with 58% for PIP joints.

No clinically significant difference in the incidence of adverse outcomes was noted among subgroups (age, weight, gender, diabetes mellitus, and location of injection) or in patients receiving multiple sequential objections.[10] Although adverse events were noted in nearly all subjects receiving collagenase injection, the incidence of major adverse outcomes was low. The majority of these complications may be categorized as self-limited, periprocedural complications, including peripheral edema, ecchymosis, injection site pain, skin tears with manipulation, and adenopathy.

Major treatment-related events included 3 subjects with flexor tendon ruptures (0.27%) and a single subject who developed complex region pain syndrome after injection (0.09%). The 3 flexor tendon ruptures were attributed to CCH injection into the flexor tendon sheath. One subject ultimately required staged flexor tendon reconstruction with a very functional outcome.[5]

Witthaut and colleagues[9] reported the combined results from 2 open-label clinical trials with 879 treated joints treated with an average of 1.2 injections per affected joint. For MP joint contractures, 70% reached full or near-full extension compared with 37% of contracted PIP joints. Clinical improvement, defined as at least 50% correction, was achieved in 89% of MP contractures compared with 58% for PIP joints.

Peimer and colleagues[11] reported the incidence of recurrence in 643 subjects previously treated in 5 clinical trials and followed for 3 years. They defined recurrence as a change from posttreatment baseline of 20° of flexion for a previously treat joint plus the presence of a palpable cord. They noted recurrence in 27% of MP joints and in 56% of PIP joints. Only 7% of recurrences had undergone some type of intervention over this 3-year period. These recurrence rates are similar to that reported in several postsurgery series.

Currently, only a single published study has ventured to quantify the long-term efficacy of collagenase injection.[12] This study followed a subset of the patients enrolled in the phase II dose-response clinical trial at 8 years after initial treatment. Recurrence was stringently defined as any increase in the degree of contracture compared with maximal extension achieved after injection. Recurrence was noted in 4 of 6 patients treated for MP contracture (66%) with an average contracture of 22°. Two patients with an average preinjection contracture of 45° had recurrence with an average contracture of 60°. No patients had chosen further intervention on the treated finger. Patient satisfaction with injection was high, with 7 of 8 patients stating that they would pursue collagenase injection for the treatment of recurrent or progressive disease.

SUMMARY

Palmodigital fasciectomy remains the gold standard. The initial outcome is, in my experience, far more predictable than either NA or enzyme fasciotomy (EF). It is also a more durable treatment. NA and EF can be conceptualized as similar procedures—one uses a needle and the other an enzyme to weaken a cord sufficient to be able to rupture it and thus straighten a contracted joint. Both are less invasive and the hand is quick to recover. Both procedures are equally initially effective. CHH seems to offer greater durability. Today's patients are often better educated and seek a specific type of treatment, in particular, effective nonoperative treatment. Pharmaceutical companies now market directly and effectively to patients, and this strategy and Internet use have already resulted in an increase in the number of patients searching for practitioners willing to administer and capable of administering collagenase treatment.

REFERENCES

1. Elliot D. The early history of contracture of the palmar fascia. J Hand Surg 1988;13:246–53.
2. Starkweather K, Lattuga S, Hurst L, et al. Collagenase in the treatment of Dupuytren's disease: an in vitro study. J Hand Surg Am 1996;21(3):490–5.

3. Desai SS, Hentz VR. The treatment of Dupuytren disease. J Hand Surg Am 2011;36(5):936–42.
4. Hentz VR, Watt AJ, Desai SS, et al. Advances in the management of Dupuytren disease: collagenase. Hand Clin 2012;28(4):551–63.
5. Zhang AY, Curtin CM, Hentz VR. Flexor tendon rupture after collagenase injection for Dupuytren contracture: case report. J Hand Surg Am 2011; 36(8):1323–5.
6. Skirven TM, Bachoura A, Jacoby SM, et al. The effect of a therapy protocol for increasing correction of severely contracted proximal interphalangeal joints caused by dupuytren disease and treated with collagenase injection. J Hand Surg Am 2013; 38(4):684–9.
7. Bendon CL, Giele HP. Collagenase for Dupuytren's disease of the thumb. J Bone Joint Surg Br 2012; 94(10):1390–2.
8. United States FDA Report: Briefing Document for collagenase clostridium histolyticum (AA4500) in the treatment of advanced Dupuytren's disease. Arthritis Advisory Committee Meeting. September 16, 2009. Available at: www.fda.gov/downloads/advisorycommittees/committeesmeetingmaterials/drugs/arthritisdrugsadvisorycommittee/ucm182015pdf.
9. Witthaut J, Jones G, Skrepnik N, et al. Efficacy and safety of collagenase clostridium histolyticum injection for Dupuytren contracture: short-term results from 2 open-label studies. J Hand Surg Am 2013; 38(1):2–11.
10. Raven RB 3rd, Kushner H, Nguyen D, et al. Analysis of efficacy and safety of treatment with collagenase clostridium histolyticum among subgroups of patients with dupuytren contracture. Ann Plast Surg 2013. [Epub ahead of print].
11. Peimer CA, Blazar P, Coleman S, et al. Dupuytren contracture recurrence following treatment with collagenase clostridium histolyticum (CORDLESS study): 3-year data. J Hand Surg Am 2013;38(1): 12–22.
12. Watt AJ, Curtin CM, Hentz VR. Collagenase injection as nonsurgical treatment of Dupuytren's disease: 8-year follow-up. J Hand Surg Am 2010; 35(4):534–9.

Needle Aponeurotomy for the Treatment of Dupuytren's Disease

Roberto Diaz, MD[a], Catherine Curtin, MD[b,*]

KEYWORDS

- Dupuytren's disease • Percutaneous needle aponeurotomy • Palmar fasciectomy
- Collagenase injection • Limited fasciectomy

KEY POINTS

- Needle aponeurotomy is a safe, effective treatment of Dupuytren's disease.
- Needle aponeurotomy can be used on multiple cords in one setting.
- Recurrence rates after needle aponeurotomy appear higher than with other techniques.

Videos of a needle being inserted into an abductor digiti minimi cord and manipulation of a pretendinous cord accompany this article at http://www.hand.theclinics.com/

INTRODUCTION: NATURE OF THE PROBLEM

Dupuytren's disease is a benign fibroproliferative disorder of the palmar fascia that can result in severe flexion contractures, significantly impairing hand function. It typically presents in the sixth decade of life, with an increased prevalence among northern European Caucasians.[1] It affects more men than women, with a male to female ratio of 3:1.[2] It is considered a genetic disease, with an autosomal dominant inheritance pattern with variable penetrance.[3] Although it can affect any digit, it most frequently involves the ring finger and small finger. Swiss physician Felix Platter first described the disease in a case report in 1614.[1] However, he mistakenly recognized the abnormality as occurring in the flexor tendons. In 1777, Englishman Henry Cline correctly described the disease as originating from the longitudinal fibers of the palmar fascia. The disease was later named after the French physician Baron Guillaume Dupuytren's, who widely studied and lectured on the disease.[1]

Dupuytren's disease causes pathologic changes among normal anatomic structures in the hand. The normal longitudinal fibers of the palmar fascia, referred to as a band, become thickened and contract into diseased tissue referred to as cord. Histologic studies of diseased palmar fascia have shown an increased number of fibroblast cells that differentiate into myofibroblasts responsible for the contractures seen at the metacarpophalangeal (MP) and proximal interphalangeal (PIP) joints.[4,5]

There is currently no known cure for Dupuytren's disease. Therefore, treatment is aimed at improving hand function through correction of hand contractures. Because the severity and rate of progression of Dupuytren's disease vary within individuals, there are many factors to consider when recommending treatment of this disease. Hindocha and colleagues[6] described features in patients with Dupuytren's disease diathesis associated with an increased rate of recurrence after

[a] Orthopaedics Department, Stanford University, 450 Broadway Street Pavillion C, MC 6342, Redwood City, CA 94063, USA; [b] Surgery Department, Palo Alto Veterans Hospital, Suite 400, 770 Welch Road, Palo Alto, CA 94304, USA
* Corresponding author.
E-mail address: curtincatherine@yahoo.com

Hand Clin 30 (2014) 33–38
http://dx.doi.org/10.1016/j.hcl.2013.09.005

treatment with palmar fasciectomy. The presence of positive family history, bilateral disease, ectopic lesions, male gender, and age of onset younger than 50 years increased the risk of recurrence to 71%, compared with 21% in patients without any of these risk factors. Recognizing these risk factors helps the surgeon in counseling the patient on the risk of recurrence before any intervention.

Once the patient and surgeon consider that treatment of the flexion contracture is the appropriate next step, there are various possible treatment options, including radical fasciectomy, limited fasciectomy (LF), percutaneous needle aponeurotomy (PNA), and enzymatic fasciectomy with collagenase injections. At present the most widely used treatment for Dupuytren's contractures is LF, which is considered the gold standard. PNA has recently gained popularity because it is a minimally invasive technique that can be performed under local anesthesia.[7] Surgeon and anatomist Sir Astley Cooper first described PNA treatment of Dupuytren's contracture in 1822.[8] The PNA technique was later modified and repopularized by French rheumatologists Lermusiaux and Debeyre in 1979.[9,10] At present, PNA is an acceptable and widely used treatment method for primary Dupuytren's contracture, and its use is expanding to include treatment of recurrent disease.[11]

Smith[12] described 3 goals of treatment for Dupuytren's contracture: (1) to significantly improve functional capability of the affected hand, (2) to reduce deformity, and (3) to prevent recurrence. Recurrence of contracture is particularly problematic because revision surgery is associated with a high rate of digital nerve injuries. Thus one philosophy in the treatment of Dupuytren's disease is to perform less invasive treatments initially, and delay the first open surgical treatment for as long as possible. PNA provides a satisfactory and less invasive treatment of appropriate cords.

INDICATIONS AND CONTRAINDICATIONS

PNA is a simple, efficient technique for Dupuytren's contractures, which can have high success and patient satisfaction. The surgeon should be capable of performing several different types of treatments for Dupuytren's contractures, and thus tailor treatment to best fit each patient. Our view of the advantages and disadvantages of available treatments of Duputyren's contractures are summarized in **Table 1**.

Regardless of treatment choice, intervention is generally recommended for patients with an MP joint contracture of 30° or greater, or any degree of PIP joint contracture resulting in functional limitations.[12] Indications and contraindications for PNA are summarized in **Table 2** . Most patients with palpable cords causing contractures are candidates for this technique. The surgeon should discuss the pros and cons and tailor the appropriate treatment to each person's desires.

SURGICAL TECHNIQUE AND PROCEDURE

The technique described here is the authors' preferred technique. The authors perform PNA under local anesthesia in a procedure room, which allows the patient to provide feedback if the needle touches the digital nerve. Others have described performing multiple needle aponeurotomies in the operating room under anesthesia.

Preoperative Planning

The surgeon should perform a full history and physical examination, taking care to document the degree of flexion contracture and the character of the disease (ie, discrete cords or nodular disease).

Before beginning, the patient is counseled to tell the surgeon if at any time he or she feels "electrical shocks" in the finger. The patient is also warned of the possibility of skin tears.

Table 1
Available treatments: advantages and disadvantages

	Needle Aponeurotomy	Surgical Fasciectomy	Collagenase Injection
Cost	Low	High	High
Recurrence	High	Low	Medium[a]
Patient inconvenience	Low	High	Medium
No. of cords that can be treated in 1 visit	Many	Many	One
Anesthesia	Local[b]	Regional/general	Local
Exposure/visualization	Blind	Open	Blind

[a] Still not clear, but early data suggest that collagenase may have fairly durable results: 35% recurrence at 3 years.[13]
[b] Some surgeons who perform extensive PNA perform the procedure under anesthesia.

Table 2
Indications and contraindications for PNA

Indications	Contraindications
Palpable discrete cord	Large, bulky, ill-defined disease (relative)
Metacarpophalangeal joint contracture >30°	Recurrent cord after surgery (relative)
Proximal interphalangeal joint contracture of any severity	Patient unable to tolerate local procedure
Elderly/frail patient	Stretchy cord that allows for full passive extension of finger
—	Uncooperative or cognitively impaired patient

Preparation and Patient Positioning

The patient is supine with the arm on a hand table. The hand is prepped and field drapes are placed around the hand.

Surgical Approach

The instillation of local anesthetic is a key part of this technique. The targeted area is marked on the skin, this being the area where the cord is most clearly palpable (**Fig. 1**). Plain lidocaine is placed just subdermally above the palpable cord. The Dupuytren's cord does not have pain receptors and, thus, anesthetizing only the overlying skin is required. This placement of the anesthetic ensures that the digital nerve is not blocked, so that the patient can warn the surgeon if the needle touches the nerve. Throughout the procedure the surgeon tests each digital nerve's sensibility by brushing a finger along each side of the fingertip and asking the patient if it feels "numb." It can often be advantageous to start with the more distal disease, so that the surgeon can move more proximally if the distal digital nerve inadvertently becomes anesthetized. The authors consider that having a sensate nerve and an awake patient helps prevent digital nerve injury.

Surgical Procedure

Step 1

The assistant pulls the finger into extension, which allows the pathologic cord to displace volarly and makes it more palpable.

Step 2

A 25-gauge needle is used to perforate the cord in the area previously anesthetized. The authors prefer to perform multiple perforations through the volar aspect of the cord along the cord's longitudinal access in an area about 1 cm in length (**Fig. 2**). These perforations do not go fully through the cord, which reduces the risk of injury to deeper structures. This technique relies on tactile feedback. The surgeon needs to feel for the diseased cord to place the perforations. The surgeon should also feel the needle "grating" as it perforates the diseased tissue (Video 1). If there is no grating, the needle should be repositioned. Others have advocated using a larger needle and to "saw" the cord, but the authors are of the opinion that this might increase the risk of injury.

Step 3

After the perforations, the finger is firmly extended to attempt rupture of the cord. This manipulation is a smooth motion whereby the palm is stabilized with one hand while the other hand straightens the finger. Often a "pop" is heard, and the patient should be forewarned (Video 2).

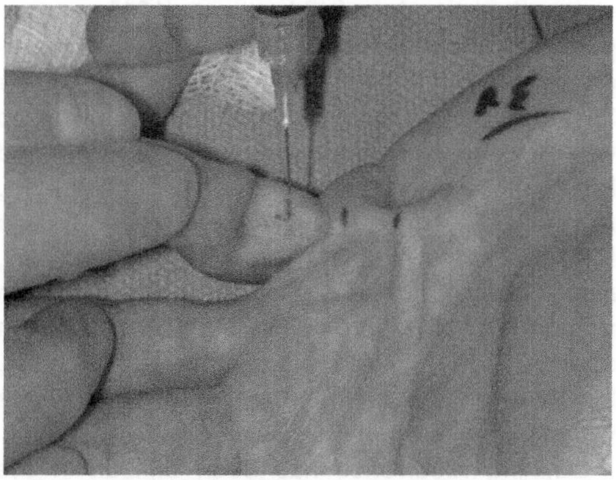

Fig. 1. Local needle being placed subdermally.

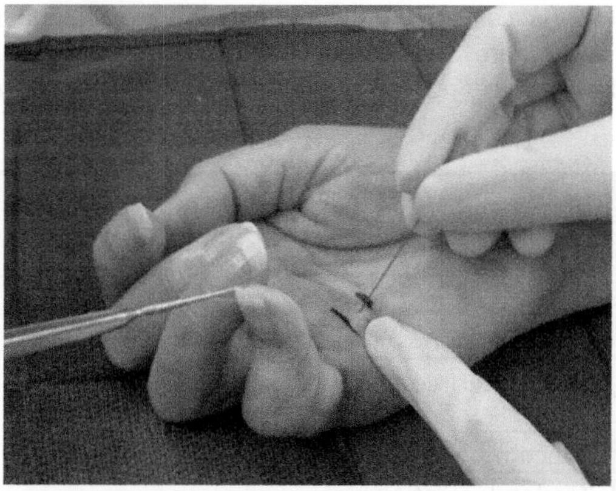

Fig. 2. 25-Gauge needle prepared for perforation.

Step 4
The assistant again extends the finger, and the surgeon palpates for any residual cords that need to be addressed.

Step 5
Step 4 is repeated as needed to achieve full extension of finger.

COMPLICATIONS AND MANAGEMENT

The complications related to treatment with PNA may be classified as major or minor (**Table 3**). Major complications include vascular injury, nerve laceration, infection, or tendon laceration. Skin tears and paresthesias that fully recover are classified as minor complications.

Several investigators have reviewed their case series and have described their results and complications. Foucher and colleagues[10] looked at 311 patients treated with PNA and found no infections or tendon injuries. Four patients experienced paresthesias and 2 had a positive Tinel sign, all of which resolved over time. One patient had persistent paresthesias after the procedure. Van Rijssen and Werker[14] reported no tendon ruptures and only 2 patients with decreased sensation in their series of 52 patients with 74 rays.

Pess and colleagues[15] provided a detailed review of their results of PNA on 474 patients (1013 rays). All patients had at least 1 MP or PIP joint flexion contracture greater than 20°. The mean preprocedure MP and PIP joint contractures were 35° and 50°, respectively. Minimum follow-up was 3 years. Complications included skin tears in 34 (3.4%) patients, transient neuropraxia in 6 (1.2%), and 1 (0.1%) nerve laceration, an overall complication rate of 4%. The overall PNA complication rate is low, and most commonly minor.

POSTOPERATIVE CARE

The patient is given a Band-Aid, or a bandage if there is a skin tear. Skin tears are treated with local wound care, and heal over the following few weeks. Patients are not given restrictions and are simply advised to be sensible, and if an activity hurts to wait until it becomes nonpainful. The authors do not routinely prescribe postprocedure therapy.

Table 3
Complications of PNA

Major	Minor
Vascular injury	Skin tears
Nerve laceration	Paresthesias with full recovery
Infection	—
Tendon laceration	—

OUTCOMES

Because there is no cure for Dupuytren's disease, recurrence is likely to occur despite surgical treatment. As such, PNA has become an attractive treatment option because it provides a less invasive first line of treatment in a disease likely to recur. This procedure can thus be thought of as a temporizing procedure that can be performed periodically to correct contractures. PNA is also a good treatment option for patients with increased comorbidities who cannot tolerate general or regional anesthesia. PNA has also been described in patients with recurrent contractures after previously undergoing LF.[11]

The outcomes of most series have looked at initial improvement and the durability of the results. Foucher and colleagues[10] reported on 211 patients who had a preoperative total passive extension deficit (TPED) of 65° that immediate postoperatively was 15°, indicating a 76% improvement in extension. A subgroup of 100 patients available for a mean follow-up of 3.2 years revealed a recurrence rate of 58%.

Van Rijssen and Werker[14] reported their early results of PNA in the treatment of 54 patients (74 rays) with an MP or PIP joint contracture of at least 20°. The mean preoperative TPED deficit was 62°, compared with 18° immediately postoperatively, a 71% improvement in extension. Thirty-eight patients (55 rays) were available for final follow-up at a mean of 33 months, 15 of whom required repeat surgical treatment for recurrent disease. Twenty-three patients did not require further surgery and had a mean TPED of 26° at final follow-up. The recurrence rate in this series was 65%. Although not statistically significant, there was a trend toward better results with lower Tubiana stages. In the series of 474 patients (1013 rays) reported by Pess and colleagues,[15] the mean preprocedure MP and PIP joint contractures were 35° and 50°, respectively. Minimum follow-up was 3 years. Immediate postprocedure MP and PIP joint contractures measured 1° and 6°, respectively. At final follow-up, the mean MP and PIP joint contractures measured 11° and 35°, respectively. Correction was better maintained in a subgroup of patients older than 55 years.[15] In summary, PNA has a high immediate efficacy, but recurrence is seen in the majority of patients within a few years.

Defining recurrence has been difficult in the study of Dupuytren's disease and its treatment.

For PNA, published recurrence rates range anywhere from 12% to 100%.[16] This variation is largely due to nonstandardized definitions of recurrence and different lengths of follow-up. Patient factors such as age at presentation and severity of disease are also likely to contribute to these wide variations. Werker and colleagues[16] performed a systematic review of 218 articles and illustrated the difficulty in reporting recurrence rates and comparing outcomes of different surgical techniques, largely because of the factors previously mentioned. Recurrence rates for patients treated with fasciectomy ranged from 12% to 73% while those treated with aponeurotomy ranged from 33% to 100%. Despite the wide range of variation in recurrence rates, this article highlights the importance of informing patients that recurrent rates are high, and appear to be higher with PNA.

Patient satisfaction is another measure that is becoming increasingly important. In 2012, Van Rijssen and colleagues[17] performed a prospective randomized trial comparing PNA with LF in 93 patients. The follow-up period was 5 years. One hundred twenty-five rays were treated with LF and 167 rays were treated with PNA. Patient satisfaction was measured on a scale of 1 to 10 (1 = not satisfied, 10 = excellent). The average satisfaction score was 8.3 for the LF group and 6.2 for the PNA group ($P = .008$). Recurrence was defined as a TPED of at least 30°. At the final follow-up, the recurrence rate in the PNA group was 85%, compared with 21% in the LF group. The investigators concluded that PNA is an effective treatment for elderly patients with Tubiana stages I and II who desire a less invasive procedure with faster recovery at the expense of increased rates of recurrence.

Needle aponeurotomy can be performed in the setting of the clinic or procedure room under local anesthesia, making PNA a minimally invasive technique with low inconvenience to patients. One comparative study of the cost-effectiveness of various treatments has favored PNA for the treatment of Dupuytren's disease.[18] In this study, the total PNA expense included anesthesia costs and hand therapy costs (neither of which the authors routinely use). Therefore, for the simple MP cord treated with PNA in the office, the costs to the health care system are far less than for the other options.

SUMMARY

PNA is one of many treatments available for the treatment of hand contractures resulting from Dupuytren's disease. It is generally recommended for elderly patients with less severe contractures who desire a less invasive procedure, or as a first stage to delay surgery in those with more aggressive disease. The procedure is safe and easily tolerated by patients, but there is a high rate of recurrence.

SUPPLEMENTARY DATA

Videos related to this article can be found at http://dx.doi.org/10.1016/j.hcl.2013.09.005.

REFERENCES

1. Bayat A, Thomas A, Warwick D. Dupuytren disease: overview of a common connective tissue disease with a focus on emerging treatment options. Int J Clin Rheumtol 2012;7:309.
2. Geoghegan JM, Forbes J, Clark DI, et al. Dupuytren disease risk factors. J Hand Surg Br 2004;29(5): 423–6.
3. Hu FZ, Nystrom A, Ahmed A, et al. Mapping of an autosomal dominant gene for Dupuytren contracture to chromosome 16q in a Swedish family. Clin Genet 2005;68(5):424–9.
4. Luck JV. Dupuytren contracture: a new concept of the pathogenesis correlated with surgical management. J Bone Joint Surg Am 1959;41(4):635–64.
5. Tomasek JJ, Gabbiani G, Hinz B, et al. Myofibroblasts and mechano-regulation of connective tissue remodeling. Nat Rev Mol Cell Biol 2002;3:349–63.
6. Hindocha S, Stanley JK, Watson S, et al. Dupuytren diathesis revisited: evaluation of prognostic indicators for risk of disease recurrence. J Hand Surg 2006;31:1626–34.
7. Desai SS, Hentz VR. The treatment of Dupuytren disease. J Hand Surg 2011;36:936–42.
8. Hutchison RL, Rayan MG. Astley Cooper: his life and surgical contributions. J Hand Surg 2011;36: 316–20.
9. Lermusiaux JL, Debeyre N. Le traitement médical de la maladie de Dupuytren. In: de Sèze S, Ryckewaert A, Kahn MF, et al, editors. L'actualité rhumatologique 1979. Paris: Expansion Scientifique Française; 1980. p. 338–43.
10. Foucher G, Medina J, Navarro R. Percutaneous needle aponeurotomy. Complications and results. Chir Main 2001;20:206–11.
11. Van Rijssen AL, Werker P. Percutaneous needle fasciotomy for recurrent Dupuytren disease. J Hand Surg 2012;37:1820–3.
12. Smith A. Diagnosis and indications for surgical treatment. Hand Clin 1991;7:635–42.
13. Peimer CA, Blazar P, Coleman S, et al. Dupuytren contracture recurrence following treatment with collagenase *Clostridium histolyticum* (CORDLESS study): 3-year data. J Hand Surg Am 2013;38(1): 12–22. http://dx.doi.org/10.1016/j.jhsa.2012.09.028.

14. Van Rijssen AL, Werker P. Percutaneous needle fasciectomy in Dupuytren disease. J Hand Surg Br 2006;31(5):498–501.
15. Pess GM, Pess RM, Pess RA. Results of needle aponeurotomy for Dupuytren contracture in over 1,000 fingers. J Hand Surg 2012;37:651–6.
16. Werker P, Pess GM, Van Rijssen AL, et al. Correction of contracture and recurrence rates of Dupuytren contracture following invasive treatment: the importance of clear definitions. J Hand Surg 2012;37:2095–105.
17. Van Rijssen AL, Linden H, Werker P. Five-year results of a randomized clinical trial on treatment in Dupuytren disease: percutaneous needle fasciotomy versus limited fasciectomy. Plast Reconstr Surg 2012;129:469.
18. Chen NC, Shauver MJ, Chung KC. Cost-effectiveness of open partial fasciectomy, needle aponeurotomy, and collagenase injection for Dupuytren contracture. J Hand Surg Am 2011;36(11):1826–34.

Percutaneous Release of Trigger Fingers

Edson Sasahara Sato, PhD in Orthopedics*,
João Baptista Gomes dos Santos, PhD in Orthopedics,
João Carlos Belloti, PhD in Orthopedics,
Walter Manna Albertoni, PhD in Orthopedics,
Flavio Faloppa, PhD in Orthopedics

KEYWORDS

• Trigger • Tendon • Tenosynovitis finger percutaneous • Corticosteroid • Surgical • Release

KEY POINTS

- Trigger finger should be treated first by steroid injection because of its low morbidity.
- Treatment of trigger finger with percutaneous pulley release can only be performed if there is active triggering of the finger.
- Clear understanding of the location of the A1 pulley is key to successfully performing a percutaneous trigger release.

INTRODUCTION

Trigger finger is a common condition caused by impaired tendon gliding at the level of the A1 pulley. This impairment prevents the tendon from naturally extending and returning to its initial position, often resulting in a locked finger. Several factors, including synovial proliferation and fibrosis flexor sheath, have been associated with triggering, but as yet there is no consensus in the literature regarding its etiology.[1] Notta[2] described trigger finger as a condition caused by changes to the flexor tendon itself as well as the sheath. Hueston and Wilson[3] demonstrated in an anatomic study that the spiral arrangement of the architecture of the intratendon fibers leads to the formation of nodules that form distally to the A1 pulley.

The epidemiology of trigger finger has been well studied. It occurs more frequently in women, on the dominant side, and in the sixth decade of life. The most affected finger is the thumb, although the occurrence of the trigger is also common in the other fingers.[4] The symptoms vary from a slight local discomfort to the formation of a tendon blockage, which leads to a deficit in actively extending the finger and to the finger remaining fixed in a flexed position.[5] Trigger finger also appears to be linked to other diseases, such as rheumatoid arthritis, gout, carpal tunnel syndrome, De Quervain disease, and diabetes.[6,7] Quinnell[1] classified the trigger finger using 5 types during flexion and extension: normal movement (type 0), uneven movement (type I), actively correctable (type II), passively correctable (type III), and fixed deformity (type IV) (**Table 1**). Trigger finger is one of the most common conditions encountered by hand surgeons.

There are several treatment options available for trigger fingers. Less invasive measures such as

Trial Registration: Current Controlled Trials, http://www.controlled-trials.com/, ISRCTN19255926.
The authors have no conflicts of interest or any financial interests in, or commercial associations with, any of the products or devices in this article.
Discipline of Hand and Upper Limb Surgery, Department of Orthopedics and Traumatology, UNIFESP – Federal University of São Paulo, Rua Borges Lagoa 786, São Paulo City, Cep: 04038-031 São Paulo, Brazil
* Corresponding author.
E-mail address: edsonsasahara@ig.com.br

Hand Clin 30 (2014) 39–45
http://dx.doi.org/10.1016/j.hcl.2013.08.017
0749-0712/14/$ – see front matter

Table 1
Quinnell classification of trigger finger

Type	Clinical Symptoms
0	Normal movement
I	Uneven movement
II	Actively correctable
III	Passively correctable
IV	Fixed deformity

Data from Quinnell RC. Conservative management of trigger finger. Practitioner 1980;224:187–90.

splinting and corticosteroid injections are well described. Patients may even experience spontaneous cure or a disappearance of their symptoms. However, many patients will ultimately require surgery for release of the A1 pulley.[1,5,6,8–13]

Splinting can result in resolution of symptoms. One study found a 54% resolution of symptoms in patients splinted for at least 6 weeks.[14] However, for splints to be effective they require many hours of wearing, which can be challenging for patients. A corticosteroid injection administered to the flexor tendon sheath has been demonstrated to produce good results with about 50% improvement after 1 injection.[1,6,9–13,15] However, this technique can result in a relapse rate of up to 29%, and patients are limited in the number of steroid injections they can receive.[10]

Open surgical release is the gold standard, and has a high rate of success with minimal morbidity. Recurrence and persistence can occur, often attributable to technical error of inadequate release.[16] Other complications such as painful scarring, infections, and nerve damage have been reported.[17,18] Open technique is a surgical procedure that requires an incision and appropriate surgical instruments. Given the predictable anatomy of the trigger finger, less invasive and costly measures have been sought for the treatment of trigger fingers.

The delicate tenotomy described in 1958 by Lorthioir[19] was an early description of a minimal approach to the trigger finger. Since that time many other investigators have reported good results using percutaneous release of the A1 pulley.[5,20–28] The authors performed a percutaneous release in 76 triggers fingers of 65 patients and achieved a remission rate of 96%, with 3 recurrences. There was no need to convert any intervention to the open method.[29] **Table 2** presents a literature review of percutaneous release, which reveals a high cure rate with few complications (**Table 3**).

INDICATIONS AND CONTRAINDICATIONS

Percutaneous release can be performed in patients with trigger finger of Quinnell classification types II to IV (see **Table 1**).

Percutaneous release should not be performed in a type I finger, which has a history of catching, though this is not demonstrable on physical examination (active triggering is necessary to confirm complete sectioning of the pulley). This technique should also not be performed if synovectomy or tenosynovectomy is a concern, for example in rheumatoid patients.

SURGICAL TECHNIQUE

The technique applied was proposed by Eastwood and colleagues[5] in 1992.

Anatomy

Before proceeding the surgeon must have a thorough understanding of the location of the A1 pulley, which can be determined using palmar surface landmarks. Anatomic studies indicate that the distance from the palmar digital crease to the proximal interphalangeal crease is approximately equal to the distance from the palmar digital crease to the proximal edge of the A1 pulley. Another finding is that the A2 pulley can be preserved by terminating the A1 pulley release 5 mm proximal to the palmar digital crease (**Fig. 1**). Landmarks of the A1 pulley include for the index finger the radial border of the pisiform proximally and the midline of the digit distally, and for the small finger the ulnar border of the scaphoid tubercle proximally

Table 2
Percutaneous release

Authors,[Ref.] Year	Method	Sample	Complications	Cure (%)
Sato et al,[29] 2004	Percutaneous	76 fingers	3 recurrences	96
Eastwood et al,[5] 1992	Percutaneous	35 fingers	2 partial relief	94
Ragoowansi et al,[26] 2005	Percutaneous	240 fingers	10 recurrences	94
Blumberg et al,[25] 2001	Percutaneous	30 fingers	1 recurrence	97

Table 3
Prospective randomized studies[a]

Authors,Ref. Year	Method	Sample	Complications	Cure (%)
Sato et al,[32] 2012	Corticosteroid Open Percutaneous	150 fingers	No	86 100 100
Gilberts et al,[34] 2001	Open Percutaneous	100 fingers	1 recurrence	98 100
Chao et al,[35] 2009	Corticosteroid Percutaneous	93 fingers	No	26 96
Zyluk et al,[36] 2011	Corticosteroid Percutaneous	105 fingers	No	89 100

[a] All were randomized by sealed envelopes.

and the midline of the digit distally (**Fig. 2**).[30,31] Once the location of the A1 pulley has been defined, the authors recommend that the needle be first introduced in the midpoint of the pulley.

Prep and Patient Positioning

This technique can be performed in the office setting. The practitioner will need a sterile drape, a 19-gauge needle, a marking pen, antiseptic solution, a sterile towel, and 2 mL of local anesthetic drawn up.

After the giving consent, the patient is positioned with the affected hand in supination. The palm and affected digit are prepared with antiseptic solution and the digit is exposed at a sterile surgical drape.

Surgical Approach

The A1 pulley is palpated directly over the metacarpal head, during active flexion-extension motions of the affected finger (**Fig. 3**). With a

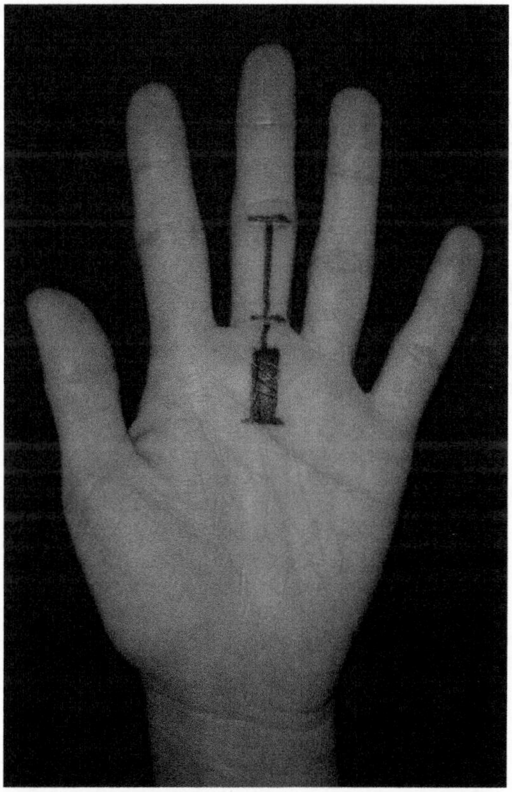

Fig. 1. A1 pulley landmark.

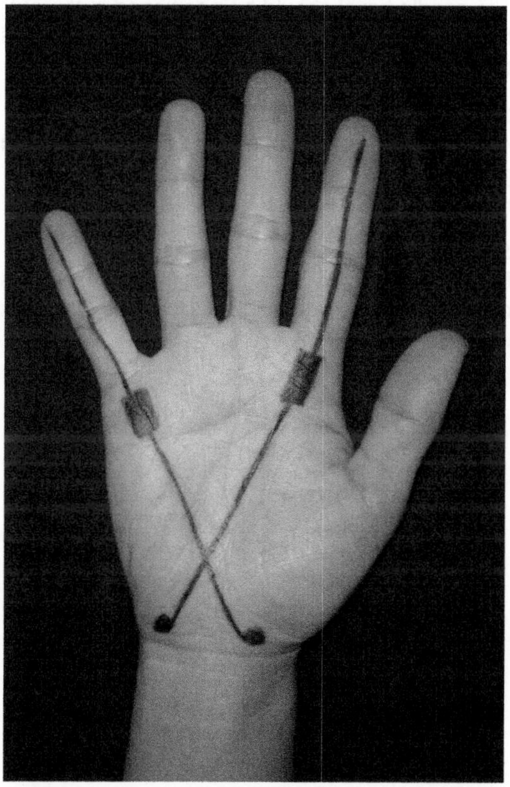

Fig. 2. A1 pulley landmarks of index and small fingers.

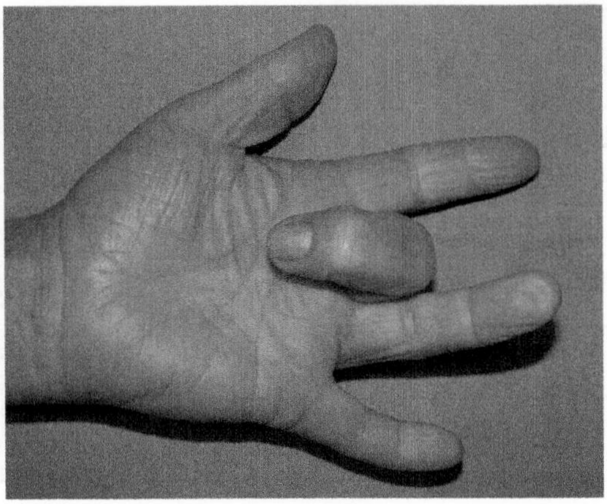

Fig. 3. Trigger finger deformity.

skin-marking pen, a line is drawn over the longitudinal axis of the digit (**Fig. 4**), and 2 mL of local anesthetic is injected into the subcutaneous tissue around the A1 pulley (**Fig. 5**).

Surgical Procedure

Step 1

The digits are hyperextended over a rolled towel to displace the neurovascular structures dorsally (**Fig. 6**).

Step 2

The needle bevel should be positioned in the cutting direction, parallel with the longitudinal axis of the digit (**Fig. 7**).

Step 3

A hypodermic 19-gauge needle is introduced perpendicularly to the skin in the site corresponding to the A1 pulley (**Fig. 8**).

Step 4

Needle placement within the flexor tendon is confirmed by finger flexion and its simultaneous displacement (**Fig. 9**).

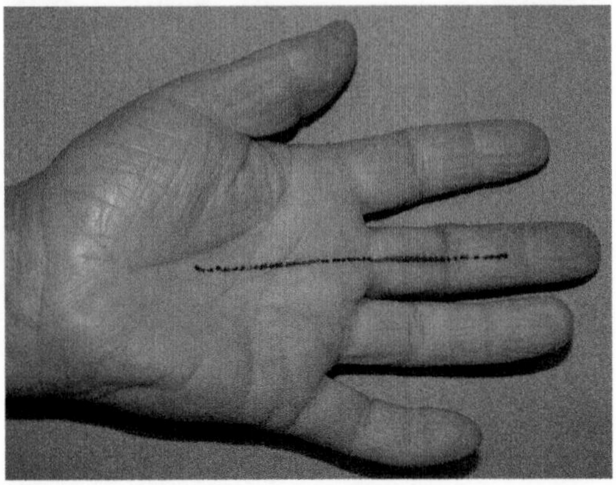

Fig. 4. Longitudinal axis of outlined digit.

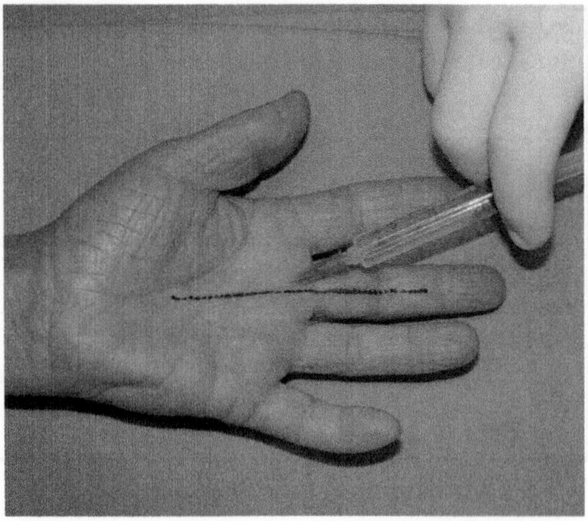

Fig. 5. Anesthetizing skin and subcutaneous tissue.

Step 5

The needle is then withdrawn slowly until removal from flexor tendon.

Step 6

Longitudinal movements of the needle are performed for A1 pulley release. Disappearance of a grating sensation indicates complete sectioning. The needle is withdrawn and the patient is asked to flex and extend the digit several times. On occasion, a second or a third needle stick distal or proximal to the initial point is necessary to complete the percutaneous procedure (**Fig. 10**). No dressings or immobilization are applied.

Immediate Postoperative Care

Free motion of the finger is authorized after the procedure, and the patient is instructed to use the hand for activities as tolerated.

Rehabilitation and Recovery

Usually there is no need for rehabilitation. If pain persists for more than 7 days, physical therapy may be indicated.

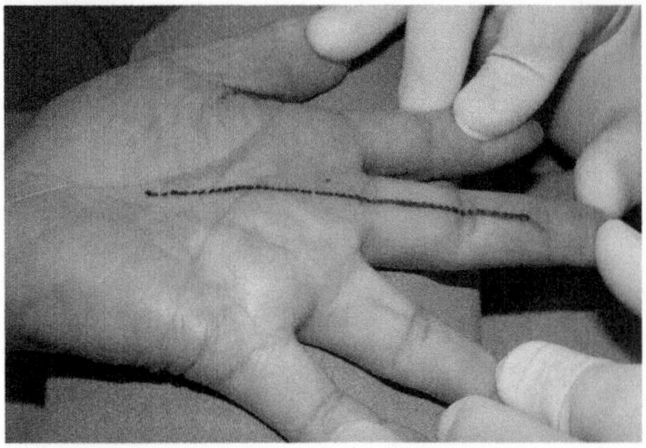

Fig. 6. Metacarpophalangeal joints in extension.

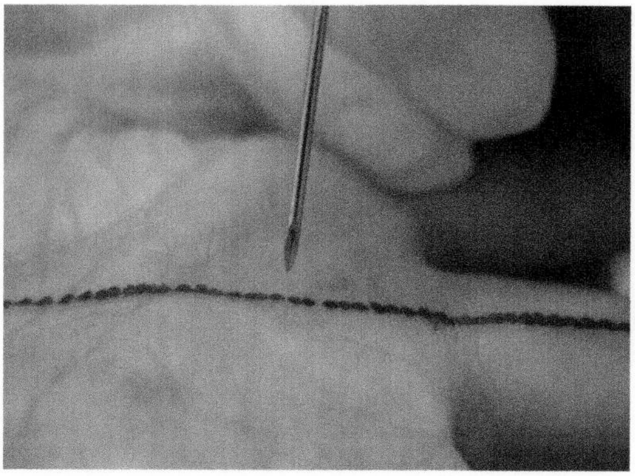

Fig. 7. Correct positioning of needle bevel during its insertion.

Pearls and Pitfalls

For trigger release, the first needle insertion should be at the midpoint of the A1 pulley. If triggering persists after the first attempt, the needle should be placed in a slightly different location, distal or proximal to the initial point. The authors believe that continued triggering after the first attempt is likely caused by proximal or distal pulley fibers continuing to catch the tendon.

The thumb is different from the fingers. For the thumb, a prominence at the palmar digital crease can be palpated; this corresponds to the flexor pulley. Usually release can be obtained by a single needle insertion.

CLINICAL RESULTS IN THE LITERATURE

The strong safety profile for percutaneous release encouraged the authors to perform a randomized prospective study comparing the efficacy of corticosteroid injection, percutaneous release of the A1 pulley, and conventional open surgery in terms

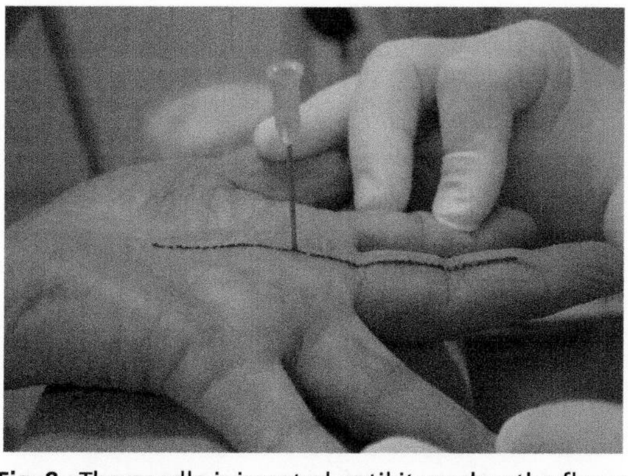

Fig. 8. The needle is inserted until it reaches the flexor tendon.

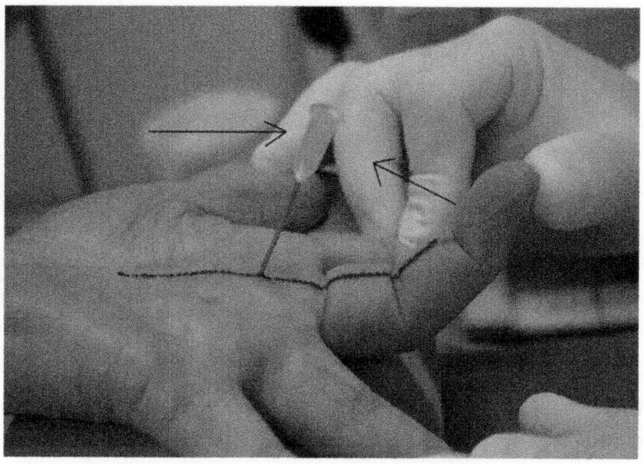

Fig. 9. Needle displacement when bending the finger.

of their rates of cure, relapse, and complications. A randomized study was performed on a homogeneous population to compare the effectiveness of these 3 methods.[32]

This trial included patients older than 15 years with a trigger on any finger. The study was different in that the authors included all fingers, whereas other studies such as that by Bain and colleagues[33] excluded the thumb and small finger because of concerns for greater risk of injury to the neurovascular bundle with the percutaneous approach. The authors included Quinnell trigger types II to IV. Type I was not included because their prior work had shown that there must be active triggering for the percutaneous method. Preprocedure triggering is required because smooth flexion-extension at the completion of the release is evidence that the pulley has been incised. With type I fingers the trigger occurs sporadically at the time of surgery and, thus, smooth gliding of the finger after release does not guarantee that the pulley has been completely released.

At the conclusion of the study, the authors found that open and percutaneous surgery had similar cure and relapse rates, and that both were superior to injection. In the injection group, a 57% cure rate of the trigger was achieved. Those who did not have relief were given a second injection, which increased the cure rate to 86% over a 6-month follow-up period. A third injection was not offered, and the relapses were considered failures. The patients in the percutaneous and open release groups had cure rates of 100%. These findings were similar to those of the randomized prospective study by Gilberts and colleagues[34] comparing the percutaneous method with the open method, in which cure rates were reported of 98% with open surgery and 100% with the percutaneous method.

The patients in the injection group experienced a lower incidence of pain in the first month of follow-up when compared with those of the open and

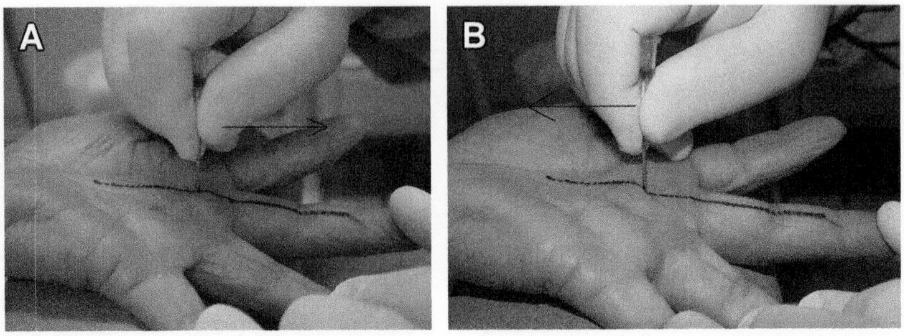

Fig. 10. (*A*) Sectioning the A1 pulley. (*B*) Sectioning the A1 pulley. (*Arrows* indicate needle displacement direction).

percutaneous groups, which had similar incidences. Investigators such as Chao and colleagues[35] and Zyluk and Jagielski[36] compared the percutaneous and injection methods, and reported that the group given injections also presented a lower incidence of pain in the first month after the procedure in comparison with the percutaneous release group. For all 3 groups, total active motion (TAM) values at the sixth month of follow-up were greater than the values observed before treatment, similar to the findings of Marcus and colleagues.[37] The open group had lower TAM values than the injection and percutaneous groups after 1, 2, and 4 months of follow-up, which may be explained by the greater morbidity of the open surgery.

The authors did not observe any injury to the digital nerve among their 3 treatment groups. The authors believe that the keys to safe percutaneous release are demarcation of the longitudinal axis of the tendon and precise anatomic knowledge of the pulleys. These tenets have been borne out in other anatomic studies.[30,31] Taylor and colleagues[38] found a complication in a 60-year-old man undergoing chronic anticoagulation therapy who presented a digital artery pseudoaneurysm following percutaneous trigger thumb release.

Percutaneous release is a blind technique that the authors have found to be safe and effective. Others have tried to use ultrasonography to allow for visualization while maintaining the percutaneous nature of the procedure.[39] The authors believe that ultrasonography adds extra expense, whereas with clear understanding the procedure can be performed without additional imaging.

SUMMARY

Open surgery has been indicated as the surgical treatment for trigger finger for many years; however, minimally invasive techniques are replacing conventional methods. Minimally invasive techniques enable early recovery of the patient with minimal damage to soft tissues. The authors' study showed that levels of effectiveness of open surgical and percutaneous methods were superior to those of the conservative method using corticosteroid based on the cure and reappearance rates of the trigger. Percutaneous pulley release for treating trigger finger is a safe, effective, and minimally invasive surgical alternative.

REFERENCES

1. Quinnell RC. Conservative management of trigger finger. Practitioner 1980;224:187–90.
2. Notta A. Research on a particular condition of tendon sheaths of the hand, characterized by the development of a nodule in the path of flexor tendons and blocking their movements. Arch Gen Med 1850;24:142–61.
3. Hueston JT, Wilson WF. The aetiology of trigger finger. Hand 1972;4:257–60.
4. Weilby A. Trigger finger. Incidence in children and adults and the possibility of a predisposition in certain age groups. Acta Orthop Scand 1970;41:419–27.
5. Eastwood DM, Gupta KJ, Johnson DP. Percutaneous release of the trigger finger: an office procedure. J Hand Surg Am 1992;17:114–7.
6. Freiberg A, Mulholland RS, Levine R. Nonoperative treatment of trigger fingers and thumbs. J Hand Surg Am 1989;14:553–8.
7. Ryzewicz M, Wolf JM. Trigger digits: principles, management, and complications. J Hand Surg Am 2006;31:135–46.
8. Patel MR, Bassini L. Trigger fingers and thumb: when to splint, inject, or operate. J Hand Surg Am 1992;17:110–3.
9. Kolind-Sorensen V. Treatment of trigger fingers. Acta Orthop Scand 1970;41:428–32.
10. Rhoades CE, Gelberman RH, Manjarris JF. Stenosing tenosynovitis of the fingers and thumb. Clin Orthop Relat Res 1984;190:236–8.
11. Marks MR, Gunther SF. Efficacy of cortisone injection in treatment of trigger fingers and thumbs. J Hand Surg Am 1989;14:722–7.

12. Newport ML, Lane LB, Stuchin SA. Treatment of trigger finger by steroid injection. J Hand Surg Am 1990;15:748–50.
13. Benson LS, Ptaszek AJ. Injection versus surgery in the treatment of trigger finger. J Hand Surg Am 1997;22:138–44.
14. Colbourn J, Heath N, Manary S, et al. Effectiveness of splinting for the treatment of trigger finger. J Hand Ther 2008;21(4):336–43.
15. Ring D, Lozano-Calderón S, Shin R, et al. A prospective randomized controlled trial of injection of dexamethasone versus triamcinolone for idiopathic trigger finger. J Hand Surg Am 2008;33:516–22.
16. Bruijnzeel H, Neuhaus V, Fostvedt S, et al. Adverse events of open A1 pulley release for idiopathic trigger finger. J Hand Surg Am 2012;37(8):1650–6.
17. Turowski GA, Zdankiewicz PD, Thomson JG. The results of surgical treatment of trigger finger. J Hand Surg Am 1997 Jan;22(1):145–9.
18. Thorpe AP. Results of surgery for trigger finger. J Hand Surg Am 1988;13:199–201.
19. Lorthioir J. Surgical treatment of trigger-finger by a subcutaneous method. J Bone Joint Surg Am 1958;40:793–5.
20. Tanaka J, Muraji M, Negoro H, et al. Subcutaneous release of trigger thumb and fingers in 210 fingers. J Hand Surg Br 1990;15:463–5.
21. Lyu SR. Closed division of the flexor tendon sheath for trigger finger. J Bone Joint Surg Br 1992;74:418–20.
22. Cohen TJ. Percutaneous treatment of trigger finger. Ver Bras Ortop 1996;31:690–2.
23. Nagoshi M, Hashizume H, Nishida K, et al. Percutaneous release for trigger finger in idiopathic and hemodialysis patients. Acta Med Okayama 1997;51:155–8.
24. Cihantimur B, Akin S, Ozcan M. Percutaneous treatment of trigger finger. Acta Orthop Scand 1998;69:167–8.
25. Blumberg N, Arbel R, Dekel S. Percutaneous release of trigger digits. J Hand Surg Br 2001;26:256–7.
26. Ragoowansi R, Acornley A, Khoo CT. Percutaneous trigger finger release: the 'lift-cut' technique. Br J Plast Surg 2005;58:817–21.
27. Wang HC, Lin GT. Retrospective study of open versus percutaneous trigger thumb in children. Plast Reconstr Surg 2005;115:1963–70.
28. Fu YC, Huang PJ, Tien YC, et al. Revision of incompletely released trigger fingers by percutaneous release: results and complications. J Hand Surg Am 2006;31:1288–91.
29. Sato ES, Albertoni WM, Leite VM, et al. Trigger finger: a prospective analysis of 76 fingers treated surgically by percutaneous release. Rev Bras Ortop 2004;396:309–22.
30. Wilhelmi BJ, Mowlavi A, Neumeister MW, et al. Safe treatment of trigger finger with longitudinal and transverse landmarks: an anatomic study of the border fingers for percutaneous release. Plast Reconstr Surg 2003;112:993–9.
31. Fiorini HJ, Santos JB, Hirakawa CK, et al. Anatomical study of the A1 pulley: length and location by means of cutaneous landmarks on the palmar surface. J Hand Surg Am 2011;36:464–8.
32. Sato ES, Gomes Dos Santos DB, Belloti JC, et al. Treatment of trigger finger: randomized clinical trial comparing the methods of corticosteroid injection, percutaneous release and open surgery. Rheumatology (Oxford) 2012;51(1):93–9.
33. Bain GI, Turnbull J, Charles MN, et al. Percutaneous A1 pulley release: a cadaveric study. J Hand Surg Am 1995;20:781–4.
34. Gilberts EC, Beekman WH, Stevens HJ, et al. Prospective randomized trial of open versus percutaneous surgery for trigger digits. J Hand Surg Am 2001;26:497–500.
35. Chao M, Wu S, Yan T. The effect of miniscalpel-needle versus steroid injection for trigger thumb release. J Hand Surg Eur Vol 2009;34:522–5.
36. Zyluk A, Jagielski G. Percutaneous A1 pulley release vs steroid injection for trigger digit: the results of a prospective, randomized trial. J Hand Surg Eur Vol 2011;36(1):53–6. http://dx.doi.org/10.1177/1753193410381824.
37. Marcus AM, Culver JE Jr, Hunt TR 3rd. Treating trigger finger in diabetics using excision of the ulnar slip of the flexor digitorum superficialis with or without A1 pulley release. Hand 2007;2:227–31.
38. Taylor SA, Osei DA, Jain S, et al. Digital artery pseudoaneurysm following percutaneous trigger thumb release: a case report. J Bone Joint Surg Am 2012;94(2):e6. http://dx.doi.org/10.2106/JBJS.K.00300.
39. Rojo-Manaute JM, Soto VL, De las Heras Sánchez-Heredero J, et al. Percutaneous intrasheath ultrasonographically guided first annular pulley release: anatomic study of a new technique. J Ultrasound Med 2010 Nov;29(11):1517–29.

Endoscopic Carpal Tunnel Release

Torben B. Hansen, MD, PhD[a,b,*],
Haider Ghalib Majeed, MD[a]

KEYWORDS

• Median nerve compression • Carpal tunnel syndrome • Endoscopic carpal tunnel release
• Minimal invasive surgery

KEY POINTS

- Minimal invasive surgery
- Effective local anesthetic surgery
- Reduces rehabilitation time
- No difference compared with open surgery after 3 months
- Operation costs higher than with open surgery
- May be more cost-effective than open surgery because of faster rehabilitation

INTRODUCTION

Nature of the Problem

Carpal tunnel syndrome (CTS) is a common compression neuropathy arising from increased pressure in the carpal tunnel. Wrist fracture, trauma, and vibration tools may lead to CTS, but in most patients the condition is idiopathic. If conservative treatment fails, a procedure to release the carpal tunnel is normally indicated.

During a carpal tunnel release (CTR), the surgeon divides the flexor tendon retinaculum, decompressing the pressure within the carpal tunnel, a technique introduced more than 60 years ago.[1] In the conventional open CTR (OCTR), the surgeon dissects directly down to the flexor tendon retinaculum through a skin incision extending from the wrist creases to the middle of the palm. The retinaculum is then split using a scalpel or scissors, resulting in decompression of the carpal tunnel. This technique necessitates an incision in the palm, which can be painful and limit recovery.

The introduction of arthroscopy for joint surgery generated the idea that arthroscopic technology could be used to treat CTS with minimal subcutaneous dissection. This idea led to the development of the endoscopic CTR (ECTR),[2] which divides the retinaculum through small portals without dissecting in the subcutaneous space above the retinaculum. Two different techniques were introduced: the 2-portal system by Chow and Hantes[3] and 1-portal systems by Okutsu[2] and by Agee and colleagues.[4] Since the initial advent, other techniques and devices have been developed, but all are variations of the original systems.

INDICATIONS/CONTRAINDICATIONS

Before any operative procedure, the first step is to ensure that the diagnosis of CTS is correct (**Table 1**). A history and physical examination often confirm the diagnosis, and the use of preoperative nerve conduction studies (NCSs) may reduce the risk of misdiagnosing symptoms

Disclosure: This work did not receive financial support.
[a] Section of Hand Surgery, Department of Orthopaedics, Regional Hospital Holstebro, Laegaardvej 12, Holstebro DK-7500, Denmark; [b] Department of Clinical Medicine, Aarhus University, Brendstrupgårdvej 100, 8200 Aarhus N, Aarhus C DK-8000, Denmark
* Corresponding author. Department of Clinical Medicine, Aarhus University, Brendstrupgårdvej 100, 8200 Aarhus N, Aarhus C DK-8000, Denmark.
E-mail address: tbhansen@dadlnet.dk

Hand Clin 30 (2014) 47–53
http://dx.doi.org/10.1016/j.hcl.2013.08.018

Table 1
Indications/contraindications

Primary Indication	Relative Contraindication[a]
Idiopathic CTS	CTS secondary to trauma/ fracture CTS associated with inflammatory disease Recurrent CTS Severe obesity Anticoagulated

[a] Consider OCTR instead.

related to other diseases, such as cervical nerve compression.

Most patients are candidates for ECTR because idiopathic CTS can be safely treated with this technique. ECTR decreases the acute morbidity after CTR, and thus, some have advocated performing simultaneous ECTR in patients with bilateral disease,[5] depending on the severity of the symptoms. Fehringer and colleagues[6] found a decrease in the time to return to work in the simultaneous group compared with the staged group, and the simultaneous group also required fewer physician visits. Overall, patient satisfaction was equal, and the use of simultaneous surgery seems to be of economic benefit to both the patient and the hospital, reducing the cost of operation and sick leave.

There are several instances in which ECTR should be approached with caution. The first group is those patients with CTS secondary to inflammatory diseases, such as rheumatoid arthritis. These patients may have synovial adhesions and hypertrophy, which can interfere with the introduction of the endoscopic device and impair the visibility in the carpal tunnel. Also, ECTR should be considered carefully in patients with a history of wrist fractures, because their previous trauma may have resulted in scarring and changes in the bony architecture of the carpal tunnel. For these patients, preoperative radiographic examination with carpal tunnel view may identify posttraumatic space-occupying changes. There has also been concern about ECTR in patients who have had a previous CTR. It is possible to perform ECTR as a revision surgery for recurrent CTS.[7–9] The most common cause of recurrence is incomplete division of the retinaculum, and this may be treated with ECTR. However, the surgeon should always consider that the cause of the failure of the previous surgery might have been a compressive lesion, such as a lipoma, an osteophyte, or an arteria mediana. These anatomic variants may not be found during an endoscopic procedure, and if they are suspected, the conventional open technique should be chosen. Also, fibrous scarring may cause compression and recurrence of CTS and should not be treated with ECTR. So, ECTR should be used with caution in recurrent cases and reserved for cases in which the patient had relief after the first surgery but had recurrence after several months. In general, the surgeon should use an open technique if any doubt exists regarding the cause of the recurrence.

ECTR should be used with care in the severely obese patient, because a large palmar fat pad may protrude into the carpal tunnel, impairing vision during the endoscopic division of the retinaculum. In addition, in the obese patient, the tourniquet may fail, resulting in a need to convert to OCTR. Another group to approach with caution is patients taking anticoagulants. OCTR should be considered for these patients, because hemostasis is easier with this technique.

SURGICAL TECHNIQUE/PROCEDURE

Preparation and Patient Positioning

The patient is placed with the arm abducted on the operation table. The surgeon is positioned so that they can use the dominant hand for maneuvering the endoscope.

Several anesthetic techniques have been described. Most commonly, the procedure is performed using local infiltration analgesia (LA) or in a regional block. General anesthesia is used only in patients who are unable to tolerate LA or block. LA is well tolerated, easy to manage, and has been proved to be more effective than a regional block, reducing costs and with less postoperative pain.[8,10]

We use the LA technique, which is simple and well tolerated. Ropivacaine 7.5 mg/mL or an equivalent local anesthetic may be used. The infiltration is performed with 4 mL administered in the proximal direction under the subcutaneous fascia of the forearm, 2 mL subcutaneously transversely in the distal wrist crease, and 4 mL subcutaneously in the palm (**Fig. 1**) along the crease between the thenar and the hypothenar. The tourniquet is then inflated to 80 mm Hg greater than systolic blood pressure 10 minutes after the administration of the local anesthetic and immediately before the skin incision.

Good visibility during the endoscopic procedure is critical to reduce the risk of complications. Using LA with epinephrine reduces the bleeding only in the skin and not in the carpal tunnel. So a tourniquet should always be used, because bleeding inevitably impairs the vision during the procedure and leads to a highly increased risk of nerve damage.

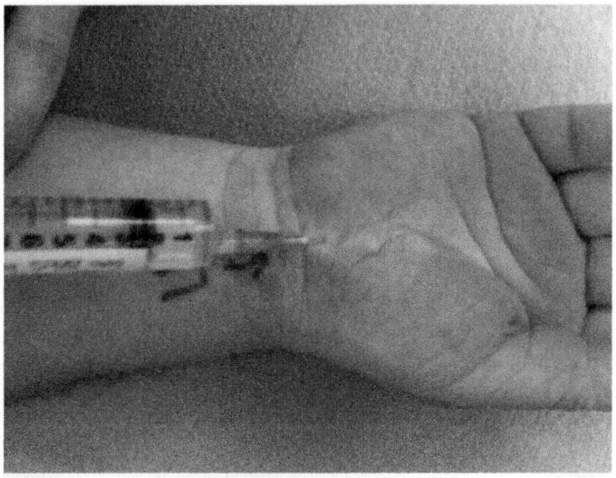

Fig. 1. Infiltrating with local anesthetics.

SURGICAL APPROACH

Because we have only a limited experience with the 2-portal technique, the following description of the operative technique is based on the Agee (Microaire, Charlottesville, VA, USA) 1-portal technique. However, apart from the difference in number of portals, the main features of the procedures are the same.

Step 1

In the 1-portal technique, the incision is a transverse incision at one of the wrist creases (**Fig. 2**). A distal hinged fascia flap is prepared, followed by clearing synovial adhesions using a dissector. This strategy allows development of a portal down to the level of the median nerve (**Fig. 3**).

Step 2

After the soft tissue is freed, the dilators are inserted. The dilators are inserted to ensure free mobility of the contents of the carpal tunnel, so that it is possible to freely move the knife above the tendons and nerve.

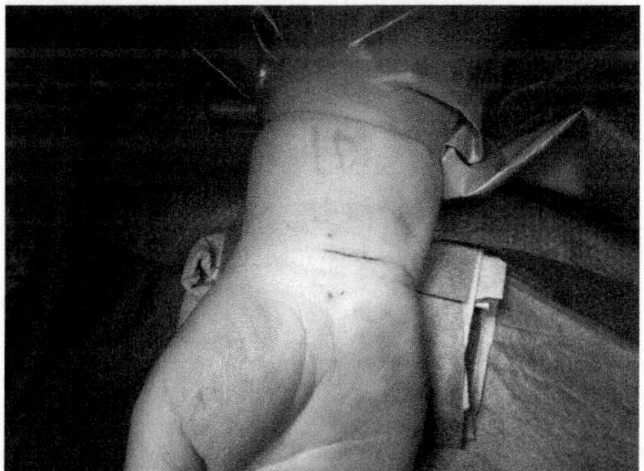

Fig. 2. Incision in the wrist crease.

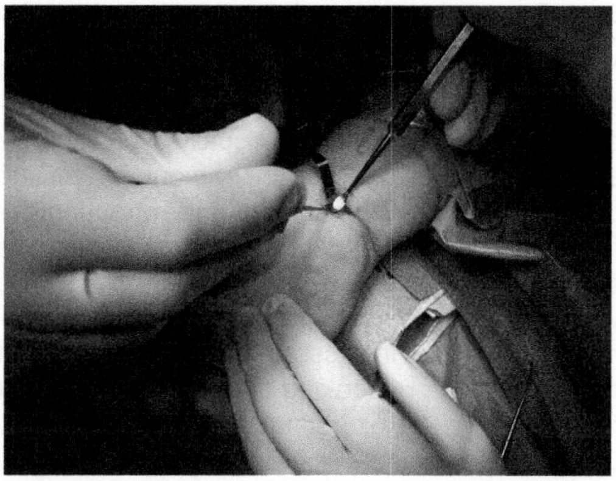

Fig. 3. Preparing for insertion of the ECTR device.

Step 3

The knife is placed so that it rests upwards onto the retinaculum oriented along the axis of the ring finger. The endoscopic knife is introduced, and the distal border of the retinaculum localized. The distal border can be visualized by a change in color and is normally well defined. If there are any problems with the visibility and the retinaculum is difficult to define, then convert to an open procedure ("if in doubt get out").

Step 4

Once the retinaculum is defined, the knife blade is engaged and the retinaculum is divided in distal-proximal direction. While drawing the knife proximally (toward the surgeon), the focus is keeping the knife in intimate contact with the retinaculum; this prevents nerve or tendon interposition (**Fig. 4**).

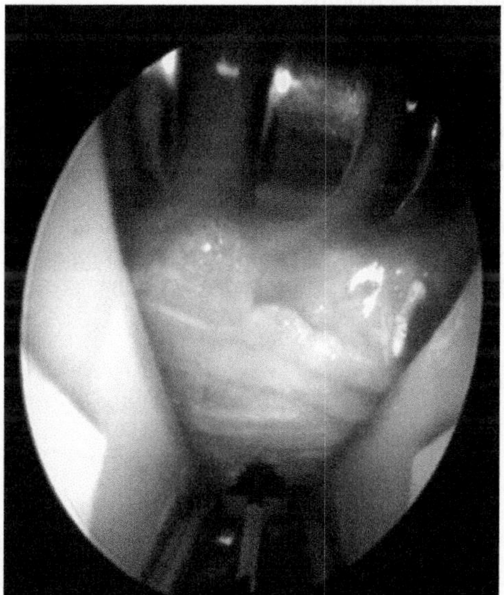

Fig. 4. The view through the ECTR device showing the knife in intimate contact with the retinaculum.

Step 5

Next, you need to ensure a complete release. To assist with this goal, we have made a special instrument by bending a hook usually used for knee arthroscopy. We use this instrument for testing the tension of the retinaculum and retracting the fad-pad (**Figs. 5** and **6**). This maneuver reduces the risk of incomplete division of the retinaculum, which may lead to recurrence of the CTS. This maneuver also helps in assessing the distal border of the retinaculum by looking for the distal holdfast fibers of the flexor retinaculum described by Okutsu.[2] These fibers tether the cut edges of the retinaculum so that it does not move freely and hang down after release. The presence of these fibers indicates that an incomplete division of the retinaculum should be suspected. In our experience, these fibers are easily assessed using the hook to test for tension and incomplete division. After dividing the retinaculum, it is important also to divide the proximal fascia edge at the portal, especially if the portal is placed at the distal wrist crease.

Step 6

The tourniquet may be deflated before the skin is sutured with interrupted nylon sutures or a continuous resorbable intracutaneous suture. After suturing the wound, additional Steri-Strips may be used. The use of intracutaneous suture may reduce pain in the first 24 hours compared with interrupted nylon sutures, but the difference is only small and the cosmetic appearance of the scar is equal after 3 months.[11]

POSTOPERATIVE CARE

The hand should be immobilized in a light compressing boxer bandage (**Fig. 7**) for 24 to 48 hours to avoid bleeding in the carpal tunnel. After removal of the large bandage, the patient needs only a Band-Aid until the wound has healed after 10 to 12 days.

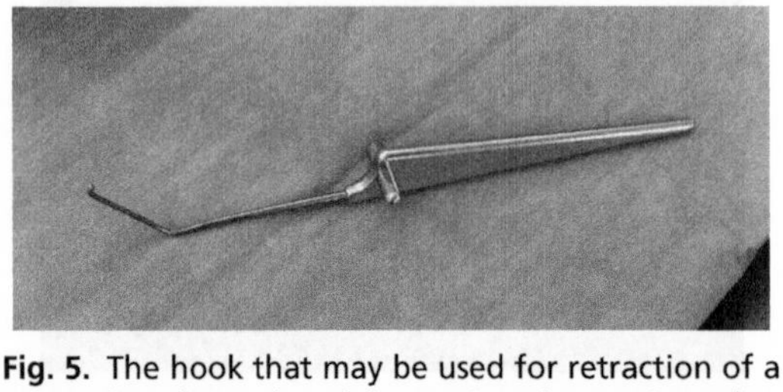

Fig. 5. The hook that may be used for retraction of a protruding fat pad and for testing the tension after dividing the retinaculum.

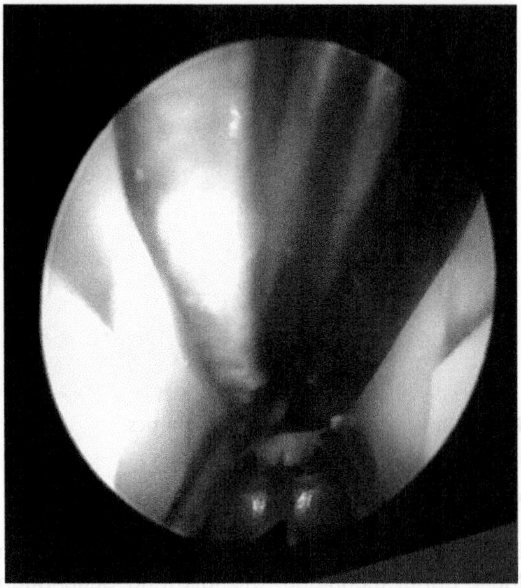

Fig. 6. The hook inserted in the carpal tunnel.

COMPLICATIONS AND MANAGEMENT

There is a significant learning curve in ECTR, but Beck and colleagues[12] found that the rates of conversion significantly diminished with increased surgeon and anesthesia experience. During this learning curve, patients may be at a higher risk of conversion to OCTR, but there is no increased morbidity. Because LA may increase the risk of impaired visibility during the procedure, it may be advised to use a regional block initially until the surgeon feels comfortable with the endoscopic technique.

The complication most feared with ECTR is injury to a nerve. Most commonly, these injuries are a transient neuropraxia. For example, decompression of the carpal tunnel using ECTR may result in changes in pressure in the Guyon canal, leading

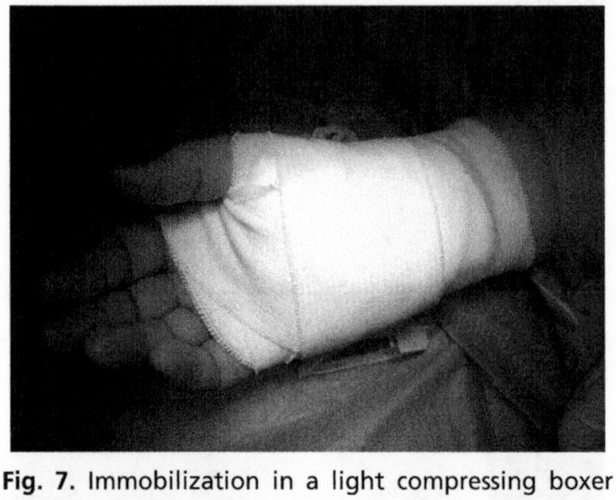

Fig. 7. Immobilization in a light compressing boxer bandage for 24 to 48 hours to avoid bleeding in the carpal tunnel.

to Guyon canal syndrome, but these symptoms are normally brief.[13] Transitory median nerve sensory disturbances also may occur after ECTR, probably because of compression, stretching, or manipulation of the median nerve during the operation. Although rare, the most serious complication is permanent nerve injury caused by cutting into the nerve.[14,15] To avoid this complication, surgeons must be aware that neural variations arising from the ulnar aspect of the median nerve are common and these could put the nerve at risk for iatrogenic injury during either endoscopic or open release.[16]

To minimize risk of complications, the surgeon must be willing to convert to an OCTR if the situation is suboptimal. In particular, the risk for nerve injury is amplified if the visibility during the procedure is impaired. Thus, if bleeding is limiting the visibility during an ECTR, the surgeon should seriously consider converting to an open procedure. Another criterion for safe release of the flexor retinaculum using ECTR is that the contents of the carpal tunnel must be freely moveable by the endoscope. If the surgeon encounters a mechanical block or significant resistance during the introduction of the endoscope (which may be caused by synovial adhesions or an abnormality within the carpal tunnel), conversion to an open procedure is highly recommended. The surgeon may also encounter difficulties when introducing the endoscope in a small wrist. Uchiyama and colleagues[17] found that tight access was experienced more frequently in younger patients and those with a small cross-sectional area at the hook-of-hamate level. These investigators found that ECTR was easily performed in older female patients. Although the younger patients were more challenging, this study did not identify a group of patients in whom ECTR should be avoided, and the conclusion was that no group should be excluded based on solely age, body size, or gender.

As with any surgical procedure, postoperative bleeding may occur after ECTR, resulting in swelling of the hand and an increased risk of infection. To limit this risk, a light compressive bandage is recommended during the first 24 hours. Also, as mentioned earlier, for patients on anticoagulants, OCTR should be considered.

Postoperative infection and reflex sympathetic dystrophy syndrome are rare complications[14,15] and not specific to ECTR compared with hand surgery in general.

Efficacy of ECTR to relieve carpal tunnel symptoms varies depending on the age of the patient, the severity of the CTS, and the duration of the nerve compression.[18–20] However, complete lack of relief of the preoperative symptoms suggests that the diagnosis may have been wrong or that there has been an incomplete release of the retinaculum. One concern with ECTR is an increase in risk of inadequate release because of limited visibility of the retinaculum when compared with the direct approach of OCTR. This risk is reduced with increasing experience with ECTR and by using our modified hook to help inspect for any residual compressive bands (see step 5). Repeat NCSs are helpful in evaluating patients who have not improved after surgery. Rotman and colleagues[21] found that postsurgical changes in the distal motor latency of the median nerve were highly dependent on the prerelease latency. This sensitivity and specificity of an NCS can aid in determining the level of improvement in median nerve function after ECTR. An NCS performed 3 months after the operation should show some improvement compared with preoperative values. If not, the possibility of an incomplete division of the retinaculum should be suspected and reoperation considered.

Overall, the literature has found ECTR to be a safe procedure. Hankins and colleagues'[14] reported on a large series of patient and had only 1 nerve injury in 14,722 patients and a conversion rate to open procedure of 0.07%. In another series of 12,702 patients, Pajardi and colleagues[15] had 6 nerve injuries (3 partial), 12 recurrences, and a conversion to open procedure of 0.46%. Benson and colleagues[22] performed a meta-analysis of 80 publications, including 22,327 cases of ECTR and 5669 cases of OCTR release, and found that the proportion of complications was very low for CTR, performed either endoscopic or open. Thus, selection of CTR technique should be based on surgeon and patient preference.

POSTOPERATIVE CARE

This section outlines our postoperative instructions after ECTR.

- To avoid wound infection, patients are advised to keep the wound away from dirt until the skin has healed after 10 to 14 days.
- Workers without hand-demanding tasks may work after removal of the compressing bandage after 24 to 48 hours.
- Workers with hand-demanding tasks may benefit from a sick leave of 10 to 14 days until the wound has healed.
- After the wound has healed, no specific restrictions are needed, and the patients are allowed to use the hand as much as pain and tenderness allow.
- Normally, no formal therapy is required.
- No routine controls are needed.

OUTCOMES

ECTR has been extensively studied. Much of the focus has been on the impact of ECTR on postoperative recovery. In this section, several randomized controlled trials that have compared ECTR with OCTR are reviewed.

Atroshi and colleagues[23] performed a randomized study of OCTR and ECTR and found that endoscopic surgery was associated with less postoperative pain, but because of the small size of the benefit, they questioned the cost-effectiveness of this improvement. In addition, they found that the median length of work absence after surgery was 28 days in both groups. However, Saw and colleagues[24] found a statistically significant difference between the 2 treatment groups, with the endoscopic group returning to work, on average, 8 days sooner than the open group. Therefore, these investigators recommended that ECTR should be considered in the employed as a cost-effective procedure, but that these cost savings may not be found in the general population. Larsen and colleagues[25] compared the results of CTR using classic incision, short incision, or endoscopic technique. They found a significantly shorter sick leave and faster rehabilitation in the endoscopic group. However, they found no significant differences in pain, paresthesia, range of motion, pillar pain, and grip strength after 24 weeks of follow-up. Kang and colleagues[26] found similar improvements in patient-reported outcome after endoscopic and open techniques at 3 months postoperatively, however, most of the patients preferred the endoscopic technique. Trumble and colleagues[27] found that during the first 3 months after surgery, the patients treated with ECTR had better CTS symptom severity scores, better CTS functional status scores, and better subjective satisfaction scores compared with OCTR. During the first 3 months after surgery, these patients also had significantly greater grip strength, pinch strength, and hand dexterity. The open technique also resulted in greater scar tenderness during the first 3 months after surgery as well as a longer time until the patients could return to work. Vasiliadis and colleagues[28] found that ECTR provides a faster recovery for the first 2 weeks, with faster relief of pain and faster improvement in functional abilities. Paresthesia and numbness subside in an identical manner with the 2 techniques. At 1 year postoperatively, both open and endoscopic techniques seem to be equivalently efficient. Macdermid and colleagues[29] found that grip strength and pain were significantly better at 1 and 6 weeks in the endoscopic group, although differences dissipated by 12 weeks and there were no other differences in outcome. Aslani and colleagues[30] compared ECTR with mini-incision techniques, and found better early satisfaction rates with endoscopic technique compared with open incision, but no difference was seen between the 2 groups after 4 months.

As stated in a recent Cochrane review,[31] "current evidence from randomized controlled trials showed that ECTR does not offer better relief from symptoms in the short- or long-term compared to OCTR, although ECTR seems to enable patients to return to their work or daily activities sooner."

However, return to work is a complex variable, and for the group of patients with workers' compensation, patient selection is an important component to a fast rehabilitation.[32] Several patient factors have been associated with work absence of more than 21 days: preoperative sick leave, blaming oneself for the hand problem, and a reduced preoperative nerve conduction of the motor branch of the median nerve to the thenar.[33] Also, other factors may help explain the large variance in the results of sick leave after CTR between studies from different countries: reimbursement systems, social factors, culture, demographic, economic, and workplace. Whatever the health system, reduced sick leave after ECTR compared with OCTR has the potential of improving the cost-effectiveness of CTR.

SUMMARY

ECTR is an elegant minimally invasive operative treatment of CTS, providing a rapid rehabilitation without increasing the risk of complications. However, there is a significant learning curve and the cost of the operation is significantly higher than with conventional open technique. However, the faster rehabilitation and the probability of reducing sick leave may lead to ECTR being overall more cost-effective than open CTR.

REFERENCES

1. Cannon BW, Love JG. Tardy median palsy: median neuritis. Median thenar neuritis amenable to surgery. Surgery 1946;20:210–6.
2. Okutsu I. How I developed the world's first evidence-based endoscopic management of carpal tunnel syndrome. Hand Surg 2010;15(3):149–55.
3. Chow JC, Hantes ME. Endoscopic carpal tunnel release: thirteen years' experience with the Chow technique. J Hand Surg Am 2002;27(6):1011–8.
4. Agee JM, McCarroll HR Jr, Tortosa RD, et al. Endoscopic release of the carpal tunnel: a randomized prospective multicenter study. J Hand Surg Am 1992;17(6):987–95.

5. Chin SH, Tom LK, Thomson JG. Does the severity of bilateral carpal tunnel syndrome influence the timing of staged bilateral release? Ann Plast Surg 2011; 67(1):30–3.
6. Fehringer EV, Tiedeman JJ, Dobler K, et al. Bilateral endoscopic carpal tunnel releases: simultaneous versus staged operative intervention. Arthroscopy 2002;18(3):316–21.
7. Jones NF, Ahn HC, Eo S. Revision surgery for persistent and recurrent carpal tunnel syndrome and for failed carpal tunnel release. Plast Reconstr Surg 2012;129(3):683–92.
8. Luria S, Waitayawinyu T, Trumble TE. Endoscopic revision of carpal tunnel release. Plast Reconstr Surg 2008;121(6):2029–34 [discussion: 2035–6].
9. Sørensen AM, Dalsgaard J, Hansen TB. Local anaesthesia versus intravenous regional anaesthesia in endoscopic carpal tunnel release: a randomized controlled trial. J Hand Surg Eur Vol 2013;38(5):481–4.
10. Nabhan A, Steudel WI, Dedeman L, et al. Subcutaneous local anesthesia versus intravenous regional anesthesia for endoscopic carpal tunnel release: a randomized controlled trial. J Neurosurg 2011;114(1):240–4.
11. Hansen TB, Kirkeby L, Fisker H, et al. Randomised controlled study of two different techniques of skin suture in endoscopic release of carpal tunnel. Scand J Plast Reconstr Surg Hand Surg 2009;43(6):335–8.
12. Beck JD, Deegan JH, Rhoades D, et al. Results of endoscopic carpal tunnel release relative to surgeon experience with the Agee technique. J Hand Surg Am 2011;36(1):61–4.
13. Okutsu I, Hamanaka I, Yoshida A. Pre- and postoperative Guyon's canal pressure change in endoscopic carpal tunnel release: correlation with transient postoperative Guyon's canal syndrome. J Hand Surg Eur Vol 2009;34(2):208–11.
14. Hankins CL, Brown MG, Lopez RA, et al. A 12-year experience using the Brown two-portal endoscopic procedure of transverse carpal ligament release in 14,722 patients: defining a new paradigm in the treatment of carpal tunnel syndrome. Plast Reconstr Surg 2007;120(7):1911–21.
15. Pajardi G, Pegoli L, Pivato G, et al. Endoscopic carpal tunnel release: our experience with 12,702 cases. Hand Surg 2008;13(1):21–6.
16. Beris AE, Lykissas MG, Kontogeorgakos VA, et al. Anatomic variations of the median nerve in carpal tunnel release. Clin Anat 2008;21(6):514–8.
17. Uchiyama S, Nakamura K, Itsubo T, et al. Technical difficulties and their prediction in 2-portal endoscopic carpal tunnel release for idiopathic carpal tunnel syndrome. Arthroscopy 2013;29(5): 860–9.
18. Yoshida A, Okutsu I, Hamanaka I. Comparison of clinical results between elderly and younger patients following endoscopic carpal tunnel release surgery for idiopathic carpal tunnel syndrome. Hand Surg 2013;18(1):59–61.
19. Nagaoka M, Nagao S, Matsuzaki H. Endoscopic carpal tunnel release in the elderly. Minim Invasive Neurosurg 2006;49(4):216–9.
20. Hansen TB, Larsen K. Age is an important predictor of short-term outcome in endoscopic carpal tunnel release. J Hand Surg Eur Vol 2009;34(5):660–4.
21. Rotman MB, Enkvetchakul BV, Megerian JT, et al. Time course and predictors of median nerve conduction after carpal tunnel release. J Hand Surg Am 2004;29(3):367–72.
22. Benson LS, Bare AA, Nagle DJ, et al. Complications of endoscopic and open carpal tunnel release. Arthroscopy 2006;22(9):919–24, 924.e1–2.
23. Atroshi I, Larsson GU, Ornstein E, et al. Outcomes of endoscopic surgery compared with open surgery for carpal tunnel syndrome among employed patients: randomised controlled trial. BMJ 2006;332(7556):1473.
24. Saw NL, Jones S, Shepstone L, et al. Early outcome and cost-effectiveness of endoscopic versus open carpal tunnel release: a randomized prospective trial. J Hand Surg Br 2003;28(5):444–9.
25. Larsen MB, Sørensen AI, Crone KL, et al. Carpal tunnel release: a randomized comparison of three surgical methods. J Hand Surg Eur Vol 2013;38(6): 646–50.
26. Kang HJ, Koh IH, Lee TJ, et al. Endoscopic carpal tunnel release is preferred over mini-open despite similar outcome: a randomized trial. Clin Orthop Relat Res 2013;471(5):1548–54.
27. Trumble TE, Diao E, Abrams RA, et al. Single-portal endoscopic carpal tunnel release compared with open release: a prospective, randomized trial. J Bone Joint Surg Am 2002;84(7):1107–15.
28. Vasiliadis HS, Xenakis TA, Mitsionis G, et al. Endoscopic versus open carpal tunnel release. Arthroscopy 2010;26(1):26–33.
29. Macdermid JC, Richards RS, Roth JH, et al. Endoscopic versus open carpal tunnel release: a randomized trial. J Hand Surg Am 2003;28(3):475–80.
30. Aslani HR, Alizadeh K, Eajazi A, et al. Comparison of carpal tunnel release with three different techniques. Clin Neurol Neurosurg 2012;114(7):965–8.
31. Scholten RJ, Mink van der Molen A, Uitdehaag BMJ, et al. Surgical treatment options for carpal tunnel syndrome. Cochrane Database Syst Rev 2007;(4):CD003905.
32. Duncan SF, Calandruccio JH, Merritt MV, et al. A comparison of workers' compensation patients and nonworkers' compensation patients undergoing endoscopic carpal tunnel release. Hand Surg 2010; 15(2):75–80.
33. Hansen TB, Dalsgaard J, Meldgaard A, et al. A prospective study of prognostic factors for duration of sick leave after endoscopic carpal tunnel release. BMC Musculoskelet Disord 2009;10:144.

Endoscopic Release of the Cubital Tunnel

Horst Zajonc, MD[a], Arash Momeni, MD[b,*]

KEYWORDS

- Cubital tunnel syndrome • Ulnar nerve • Endoscopic release • In situ decompression
- Compression neuropathy

KEY POINTS

- Although different surgical approaches exist for the treatment of cubital tunnel syndrome, in situ decompression of the ulnar nerve has been demonstrated to have equivalent surgical efficacy when compared with nerve transposition.
- The evolution toward procedures associated with less patient morbidity is reflected by the introduction of endoscopic techniques for the treatment of cubital tunnel syndrome.
- The authors have incorporated the endoscopic approach as proposed by Hoffmann and Siemionow[26] into their practice. Although the skin incision can frequently be kept to a minimum (<2 cm), superior visualization associated with this approach allows for in situ decompression of the ulnar nerve along a distance of up to 30 cm.

INTRODUCTION

Ulnar nerve compression at the elbow (ie, cubital tunnel syndrome) remains the second most common neuropathy of the upper extremity. A reported incidence of 24.7 cases per 100,000 per year translates into approximately 75,000 new cases of cubital tunnel syndrome in the United States annually.[1–3] Of note, men are affected almost twice as common as women.[2]

Cubital tunnel syndrome can be characterized as either primary (ie, idiopathic) or secondary (eg, caused by trauma, a space-occupying lesion, anomalous anconeus epitrochlearis muscle, and so forth) and is commonly staged based on the criteria established by McGowan[4] and Dellon.[5]

Despite the fact that the history of surgical treatment of cubital tunnel syndrome spans almost 2 centuries,[6] contemporary treatment recommendations are still characterized by a lack of consensus.[3,7,8] Despite the multitude of available treatment options, almost all procedures fall into one of the following 3 categories:

1. In situ decompression of the ulnar nerve at the level of the cubital tunnel[9–13]
2. Decompression with anterior transposition of the ulnar nerve (ie, subcutaneous vs intramuscular vs submuscular transposition)[10,14–17]
3. Medial epicondylectomy with or without decompression[18,19]

Although proponents of in situ decompression point out the advantages of this approach (ie, procedural simplicity, decreased operative time and morbidity with faster recovery, as well as preservation of neural blood supply[20]), proponents of nerve transposition argue that dynamic compression of the nerve with elbow flexion is not accounted for in simple (ie, in situ) decompression.[21,22] Despite the ongoing controversy, numerous investigators have demonstrated equivalent surgical outcomes after in situ decompression versus transposition;

The authors have nothing to disclose.
[a] Department of Plastic and Hand Surgery, University of Freiburg Medical Center, Hugstetter Strasse 55, 79106 Freiburg, Germany; [b] Division of Plastic and Reconstructive Surgery, Stanford University Medical Center, 770 Welch Road, Suite 400, Palo Alto, CA 94304, USA
* Corresponding author.
E-mail address: amomeni@stanford.edu

Hand Clin 30 (2014) 55–62
http://dx.doi.org/10.1016/j.hcl.2013.08.021

however, the group undergoing transposition had higher complication rates.[10–12] In fact, 2 recent meta-analyses comparing anterior transposition with simple decompression failed to demonstrate superiority of one approach over the other.[3,7] In light of equivalent surgical efficacy, it seems prudent to choose the less morbid procedure (ie, in situ release).

The trend to perform less extensive dissections is paralleled by a trend toward smaller access incisions as well as endoscopic techniques for the treatment of cubital tunnel syndrome.[23,24] The clinical concern with smaller skin incisions is that a point of compression may be missed because of the decreased area visualized. The authors think that the endoscopic approach provides for decompression of the ulnar nerve over a long distance with excellent visibility via a minimally invasive approach, thus, allowing for the benefits of a small incision and decreasing the risk of an inadequate release. This notion of maximizing benefit and reducing morbidity is supported by the results of a comparative analysis of endoscopic versus open in situ decompression, which demonstrated a significantly lower postoperative complication rate in patients undergoing endoscopic in situ decompression.[25]

In this article, the authors present and discuss their preferred approach to surgical decompression of the ulnar nerve using an endoscopic approach as proposed by Hoffman and Siemionow.[26] The authors discuss indications and contraindications for the endoscopic approach, present the surgical technique in a stepwise manner, and discuss postoperative management and rehabilitation.

PREOPERATIVE WORKUP

Before performing any surgical intervention, a thorough diagnostic workup is mandatory. In addition to obtaining a complete history and physical examination (including provocative testing, such as Tinel sign, elbow flexion, pressure provocation, and combined elbow flexion and pressure provocation[27,28]), nerve conduction studies are typically part of the initial workup. Occasionally, radiographic images of the elbow joint are obtained. Although additional imaging studies, such as ultrasound and magnetic resonance imaging, have been proposed, these modalities are not typically used in the authors' practice.[29,30]

In the absence of progressive symptoms, patients diagnosed with cubital tunnel syndrome are typically treated conservatively for 3 to 6 months. If nonoperative treatment measures are unsuccessful, patients are offered surgical intervention.

INDICATIONS AND CONTRAINDICATIONS

The ideal candidate for an endoscopic cubital tunnel release is a patient with primary (ie, idiopathic) cubital tunnel syndrome who has failed conservative treatment. Further indications include secondary exploration after previous endoscopic or open in situ decompression of the ulnar nerve.

Relative contraindications include subluxation of the ulnar nerve and a surgeon's inexperience with endoscopic techniques.[31] Absolute contraindications include space-occupying lesions (eg, tumors, osteophytes, and so forth), long-standing elbow contractures requiring release, prior trauma with extensive scar formation, and prior open decompression with transposition of the ulnar nerve.[31]

EQUIPMENT AND INSTRUMENTS

The authors use the HOFFMANN Cubital Tunnel Set (Karl Storz, Tuttlingen, Germany), which includes the following chief components:

1. 30° endoscope with a 4 mm diameter and a length of 18 cm (**Fig. 1**A)
2. Optical dissector with a distal spatula (see **Fig. 1**B)
3. Illuminated specula with blade lengths of 90 and 110 mm (see **Fig. 1**C)
4. Tunneling forceps
5. Curved Metzenbaum scissors with varying lengths (18, 23, and 28 cm)

SURGICAL APPROACH

The procedure is performed under regional or general anesthesia with the patient in the supine position. The upper extremity is placed on an arm table with the shoulder abducted and externally rotated and the elbow flexed and supinated. The surgeon is seated so as to face the medial epicondyle (**Fig. 2**). A nonsterile tourniquet is placed high on the upper arm to permit adequate surgical release proximally. The upper extremity is then prepped and draped in sterile fashion, exsanguinated with an Esmarch rubber band, and the tourniquet is inflated to 250 mm Hg (or 100 mm Hg greater than the patients' systolic pressure). Folded towels are used to elevate the elbow off of the table to facilitate instrumentation.

Step 1

An approximately 1.5- to 2.0-cm longitudinal skin incision is made along the retrocondylar groove between the medial epicondyle and the olecranon (**Fig. 3**A). Subcutaneous dissection continues using scissors in a spreading fashion so as to

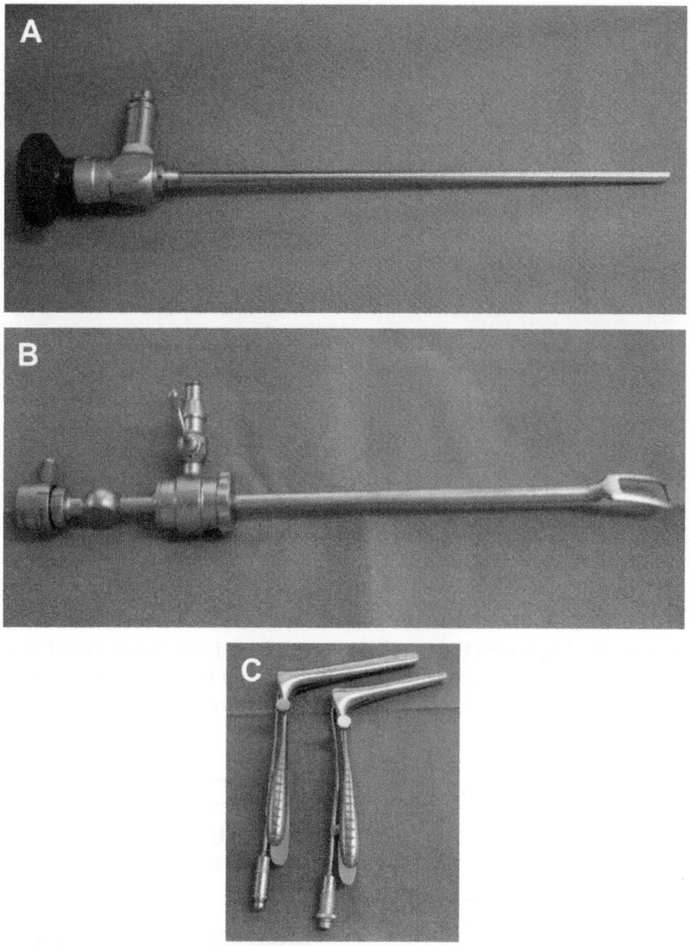

Fig. 1. Components of the HOFFMANN Cubital Tunnel Set (in addition to tunneling forceps and curved Metzenbaum scissors): (*A*) 30° endoscope with a 4 mm diameter and a length of 18 cm, (*B*) optical dissector with a distal spatula, (*C*) illuminated specula with blade lengths of 90 and 110 mm.

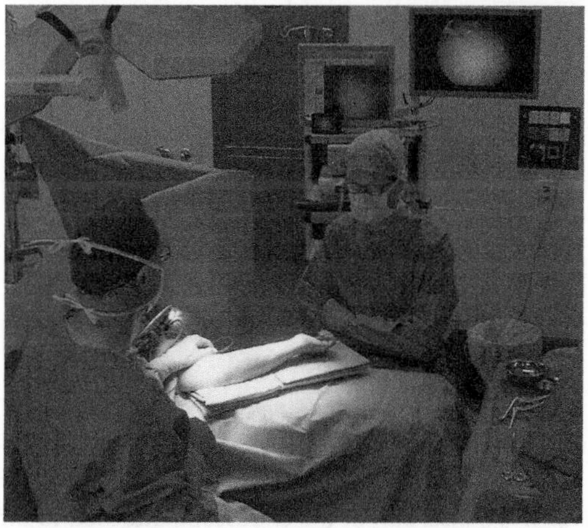

Fig. 2. Operating room setup: The operating surgeon faces the medial epicondyle, and the endoscopy tower is positioned at the head of the patient.

preserve cutaneous nerve branches until the roof of the cubital tunnel is identified. It is important to dissect straight down toward the cubital tunnel roof as opposed to creating subcutaneous tunnels by beveling proximally or distally during this step.

Step 2

The location of the ulnar nerve posterior to the medial epicondyle (ie, within the retrocondylar groove) is confirmed via palpation. Next, the roof of the cubital tunnel (ie, Osborne ligament) is divided over a short distance in its proximal aspect, thus, exposing the ulnar nerve, which is easily identified by its longitudinally oriented vasa nervorum (see **Fig. 3**B). The nerve is left in situ and not mobilized. If an anconeus epitrochearis muscle is present, as has been reported in 3.2% of patients, it has to be released as it courses over the cubital tunnel.[32] If the anconeus muscle

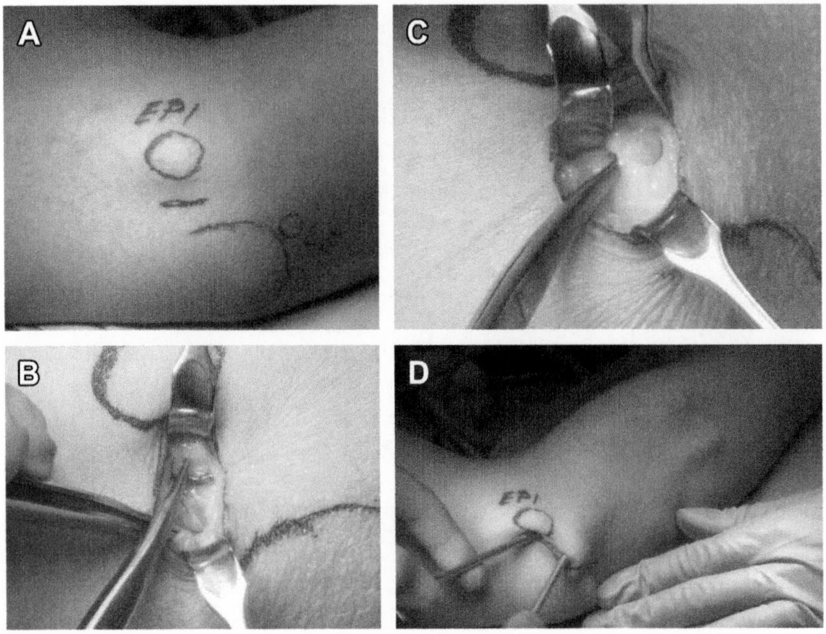

Fig. 3. (*A*) Skin incision is marked between the medial epicondyle and olecranon. (*B*) After division of the roof of the cubital tunnel, the ulnar nerve is easily identified by its longitudinally oriented vasa nervorum. (*C*) Proximal cut end of Osborne ligament. (*D*) Extent of epifascial pocket dissection.

is encountered, the incision need not be extended because the muscle is readily transected via the original incision.

Step 3

After having identified the ulnar nerve and the proximal cut end of the Osborne ligament (see **Fig. 3**C), epifascial dissection just above the fascia is performed along the course of the ulnar nerve using tunneling forceps. Dissection is directed distally toward the Guyon canal and proximally toward the anterior axillary fold. It is critical to remain epifascial because inadvertent insertion below the Osborne ligament can result in injury to the ulnar nerve. Also, it is important that the epifascial plane is created by gently spreading the tunneling forceps because abrupt maneuvers may result in bleeding and/or injury to crossing cutaneous nerve fibers. The epifascial pocket created extends approximately 15 cm distally and 10 to 15 cm proximally (as measured from the proximal border of the medial epicondyle) (see **Fig. 3**D).

Step 4

An illuminated speculum is used to visualize the distal extent of the dissection (ie, epifascial pocket). Division of the Osborne ligament is then performed under direct vision with scissors until the 2 heads of the flexor carpi ulnaris (FCU) muscle come into view.

Step 5

The endoscope attached to the optical dissector with a distal spatula is introduced, paying particular attention to staying above the fascia (**Fig. 4**A). In

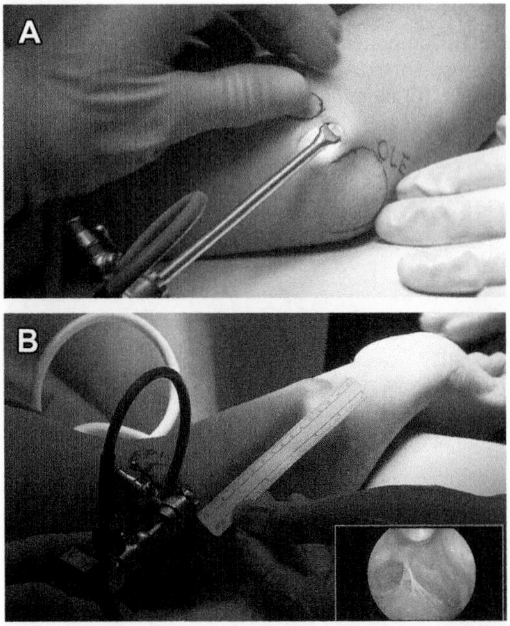

Fig. 4. (*A*) Insertion of the endoscope attached to the optical dissector with distal spatula. (*B*) Endoscope is easily advanced distally to approximately 15 cm distal to the medial epicondyle.

order to maintain adequate visibility, it is imperative to lift the dissector superficially during the procedure because this will prevent collapse of the epifascial pocket that is created. Although the dissector is easily advanced distally, fascial division is performed under endoscopic control with Metzenbaum scissors over a length of 15 cm (as measured from the proximal border of the medial epicondyle) (see **Fig. 4**B). It is critical to preserve crossing veins and sensory nerve branches during this step by lifting them off of the underlying fascia with the dissector (**Fig. 5**A). Any bleeding encountered is addressed with bipolar forceps.

Step 6

The next step involves release in a deeper layer. For this purpose, the dissector is retrieved back to the level of the skin incision and advanced again distally in a deeper layer. While advancing distally, all nerve-constricting structures are divided up to approximately 15 cm distal to the proximal border of the medial epicondyle. It is imperative to divide the deep fascial band between the 2 FCU heads (see **Fig. 5**B). After complete division, motor branches of the ulnar nerve entering the FCU routinely come into view (see **Fig. 5**C). During the dissection, any iatrogenic compression of the ulnar nerve is to be avoided. Successful dissection and in situ decompression preserves the blood supply to the ulnar nerve and frees it from all crossing structures (see **Fig. 5**D).

Step 7

Proximal release is performed in a similar fashion, with decompression of the ulnar nerve being performed over a length of 10 to 15 cm (based on upper arm length) (**Fig. 6**). Again, a stepwise approach is chosen, with division of the superficial muscle fascia initially (**Fig. 7**A), followed by release of the ulnar nerve from its investing connective tissues (see **Fig. 7**B).

Final inspection of the decompressed ulnar nerve (see **Fig. 7**C) is performed as the endoscope is retrieved.

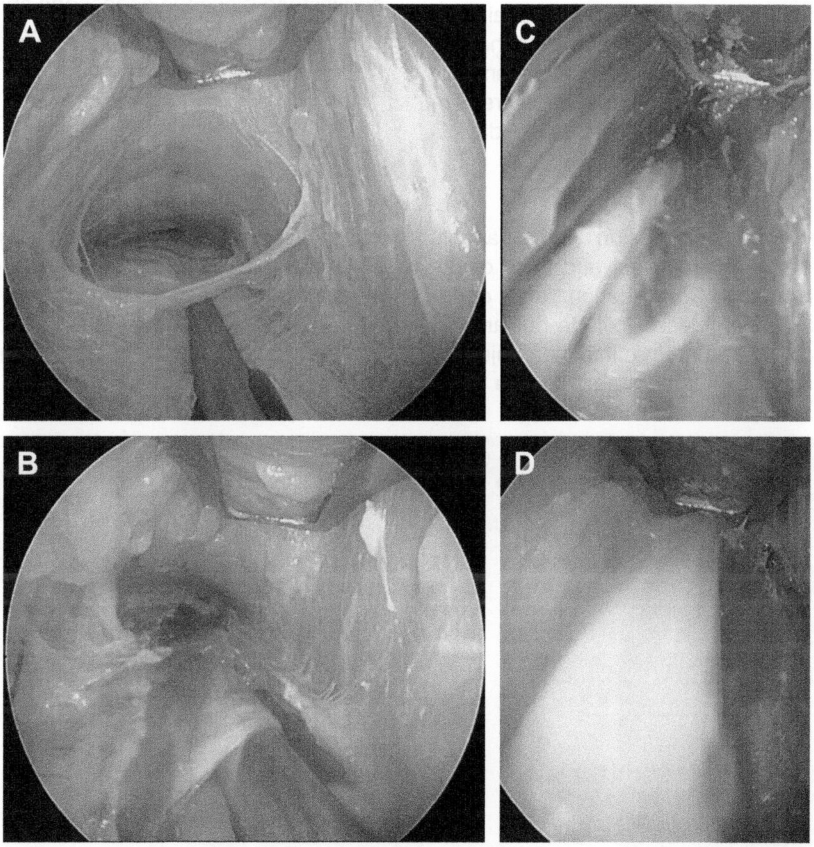

Fig. 5. (*A*) Crossing nerve fibers are protected by lifting them up with the dissector and, thus, keeping these structures out of harms way during fascial division. (*B*) The fascial band between the 2 FCU heads is divided. (*C*) Motor branches of the ulnar nerve to the FCU muscle are routinely encountered after distal release. (*D*) Appearance of ulnar nerve after completion of distal release.

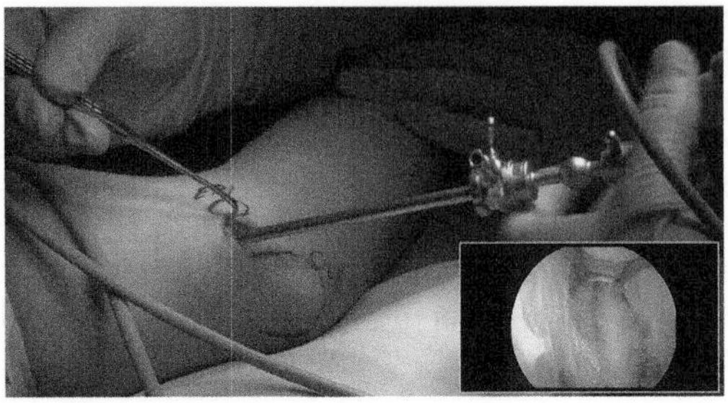

Fig. 6. Proximal release of ulnar nerve.

Step 8

Layered closure of the incision is performed, and a sterile compressive dressing is applied. The tourniquet is then deflated, and the patient is transferred to the postanesthesia care unit.

POSTOPERATIVE CARE

Patients are instructed to keep the extremity elevated in the immediate postoperative period. The compressive dressing is typically removed on the third postoperative day, with subsequent initiation of range-of-motion exercises. The goal is to have full range of motion by the end of the first week postoperatively. Return to work depends of the patients' occupation, with manual laborers generally returning back to work within 10 to 14 days.

COMPLICATIONS

Having a thorough discussion with patients regarding benefits, alternatives, and risks of the intervention is critical. Complications after endoscopic cubital tunnel release include but are not limited to bleeding/hematoma, infection, injury to adjacent structures (most notably to the ulnar nerve itself but also to the medial antebrachial cutaneous nerve), the necessity to convert to an open procedure, persistent neurologic symptoms, chronic pain/complex regional pain syndrome, and the necessity for further interventions.

OUTCOMES

Although an increasing number of investigators have published their experience with endoscopic cubital tunnel release,[33–35] an objective comparison between open and endoscopic in situ decompression of the ulnar nerve is difficult to perform. Reasons include a lack of technical uniformity, with each group using a their own endoscopic technique.[24,31,35] More importantly, proposed endoscopic techniques also differ conceptually from one another. Although most approaches involve the insertion of instruments within the cubital tunnel[24,31,35,36] (a maneuver that has been criticized because of concerns of aggravating compression of the ulnar nerve within an already-tight cubital tunnel), others have avoided blind introduction of instruments into the cubital tunnel and instead place the endoscope epifascially.[26,37]

In addition to technical variability, contemporary literature is characterized by a paucity of head-to-head comparative analyses of the endoscopic versus open approach. In a comparative analysis including 34 patients who underwent endoscopic (N = 19) versus open (N = 15) in situ decompression, Watts and Bain[25] reported higher levels of patient satisfaction with the endoscopic approach at 12 months postoperatively. Although the difference in patient satisfaction was not statistically significant, a statistically higher rate of postoperative complications was reported after open in situ decompression. Interestingly, 3 out of 15 (20%)

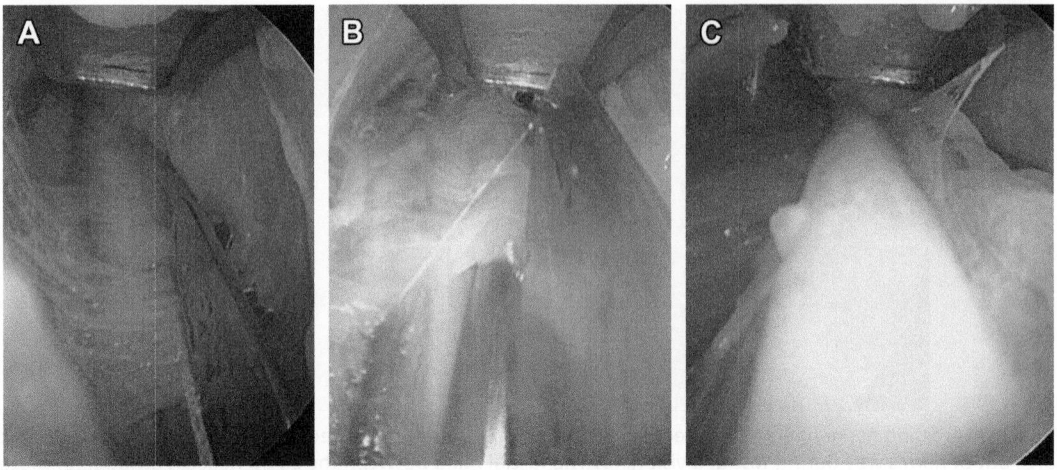

Fig. 7. (*A*) Division of superficial muscle fascia. (*B*) Release of ulnar nerve from its investing connective tissues. (*C*) Final inspection of decompressed ulnar nerve.

and 2 out of 15 (13.3%) patients complained of numbness at the elbow and scar tenderness after open decompression, respectively, whereas this was not seen in any of the patients who underwent endoscopic release. The investigators concluded that, although functional outcomes are equivalent, patients undergoing open decompression are more prone to developing postoperative complications.[25]

More recently, in a study including 114 patients, Dutzmann and colleagues[37] reported their experience comparing open (N = 59) versus retractor-endoscopic (N = 55) in situ decompression of the ulnar nerve in cubital tunnel syndrome. Although postoperative Bishop scores were not significantly different between study groups at 24 months, patients undergoing endoscopic decompression had more favorable short-term results (ie, shorter time required for return to full activity and shorter duration of postoperative pain). Similar to the observation made by Watts and Bain,[25] 23.7% of patients who underwent open decompression experienced postoperative numbness around the elbow versus none in the endoscopy group. The investigators concluded that although long-term outcomes are equivalent, short-term results are more favorable in patients undergoing endoscopic decompression.[37]

SUMMARY

It is safe to say that in situ decompression of the ulnar nerve in cubital tunnel syndrome has been demonstrated to achieve equivalent functional results when compared with more elaborate techniques, such as decompression with nerve transposition. The evolution toward procedures associated with less patient morbidity is reflected by the introduction of endoscopic techniques for the treatment of cubital tunnel syndrome. The authors have incorporated the endoscopic approach as proposed by Hoffmann and Siemionow into their practice and have obtained favorable results. Although the skin incision can frequently be kept to a minimum (<2 cm), superior visualization associated with this approach allows for in situ decompression of the ulnar nerve along a distance of up to 30 cm. Despite the extent of decompression performed, operative morbidity is minimal, with return to full duty being the rule even in manual laborers within 10 to 14 days postoperatively.

REFERENCES

1. Fernandez E, Pallini R, Lauretti L, et al. Neurosurgery of the peripheral nervous system: cubital tunnel syndrome. Surg Neurol 1998;50:83–5.
2. Mondelli M, Giannini F, Ballerini M, et al. Incidence of ulnar neuropathy at the elbow in the province of Siena (Italy). J Neurol Sci 2005;234:5–10.
3. Zlowodzki M, Chan S, Bhandari M, et al. Anterior transposition compared with simple decompression for treatment of cubital tunnel syndrome. A meta-analysis of randomized, controlled trials. J Bone Joint Surg Am 2007;89:2591–8.
4. Mc GA. The results of transposition of the ulnar nerve for traumatic ulnar neuritis. J Bone Joint Surg Br 1950;32:293–301.
5. Dellon AL. Review of treatment results for ulnar nerve entrapment at the elbow. J Hand Surg Am 1989;14:688–700.
6. Bartels RH. History of the surgical treatment of ulnar nerve compression at the elbow. Neurosurgery 2001;49:391–9 [discussion: 399–400].
7. Macadam SA, Gandhi R, Bezuhly M, et al. Simple decompression versus anterior subcutaneous and submuscular transposition of the ulnar nerve for cubital tunnel syndrome: a meta-analysis. J Hand Surg Am 2008;33:1314.e1311–2.
8. Macadam SA, Bezuhly M, Lefaivre KA. Outcomes measures used to assess results after surgery for cubital tunnel syndrome: a systematic review of the literature. J Hand Surg Am 2009;34:1482–91.e5.
9. Bartels RH, Menovsky T, Van Overbeeke JJ, et al. Surgical management of ulnar nerve compression at the elbow: an analysis of the literature. J Neurosurg 1998;89:722–7.
10. Bartels RH, Verhagen WI, van der Wilt GJ, et al. Prospective randomized controlled study comparing simple decompression versus anterior subcutaneous transposition for idiopathic neuropathy of the ulnar nerve at the elbow: part 1. Neurosurgery 2005;56:522–30 [discussion: 522–30].
11. Biggs M, Curtis JA. Randomized, prospective study comparing ulnar neurolysis in situ with submuscular transposition. Neurosurgery 2006;58:296–304 [discussion: 296–304].
12. Nabhan A, Ahlhelm F, Kelm J, et al. Simple decompression or subcutaneous anterior transposition of the ulnar nerve for cubital tunnel syndrome. J Hand Surg Br 2005;30:521–4.
13. Waugh RP, Zlotolow DA. In situ decompression of the ulnar nerve at the cubital tunnel. Hand Clin 2007;23:319–27, vi.
14. Krishnan KG, Pinzer T, Schackert G. A novel endoscopic technique in treating single nerve entrapment syndromes with special attention to ulnar nerve transposition and tarsal tunnel release: clinical application. Neurosurgery 2006;59:ONS89–100 [discussion: ONS89–100].
15. Davis GA, Bulluss KJ. Submuscular transposition of the ulnar nerve: review of safety, efficacy and correlation with neurophysiological outcome. J Clin Neurosci 2005;12:524–8.

16. Leone J, Bhandari M, Thoma A. Anterior intramuscular transposition with ulnar nerve decompression at the elbow. Clin Orthop Relat Res 2001;132–9.
17. Dellon AL, Coert JH. Results of the musculofascial lengthening technique for submuscular transposition of the ulnar nerve at the elbow. J Bone Joint Surg Am 2004;86(Suppl 1):169–79.
18. Dinh PT, Gupta R. Subtotal medial epicondylectomy as a surgical option for treatment of cubital tunnel syndrome. Tech Hand Up Extrem Surg 2005;9:52–9.
19. Efstathopoulos DG, Themistocleous GS, Papagelopoulos PJ, et al. Outcome of partial medial epicondylectomy for cubital tunnel syndrome. Clin Orthop Relat Res 2006;444:134–9.
20. Heithoff SJ. Cubital tunnel syndrome does not require transposition of the ulnar nerve. J Hand Surg Am 1999;24:898–905.
21. Kleinman WB. Cubital tunnel syndrome: anterior transposition as a logical approach to complete nerve decompression. J Hand Surg Am 1999;24:886–97.
22. Macnicol MF. The results of operation for ulnar neuritis. J Bone Joint Surg Br 1979;61:159–64.
23. Taniguchi Y, Takami M, Takami T, et al. Simple decompression with small skin incision for cubital tunnel syndrome. J Hand Surg Br 2002;27:559–62.
24. Tsai TM, Chen IC, Majd ME, et al. Cubital tunnel release with endoscopic assistance: results of a new technique. J Hand Surg Am 1999;24:21–9.
25. Watts AC, Bain GI. Patient-rated outcome of ulnar nerve decompression: a comparison of endoscopic and open in situ decompression. J Hand Surg Am 2009;34:1492–8.
26. Hoffmann R, Siemionow M. The endoscopic management of cubital tunnel syndrome. J Hand Surg Br 2006;31:23–9.
27. Novak CB, Lee GW, Mackinnon SE, et al. Provocative testing for cubital tunnel syndrome. J Hand Surg Am 1994;19:817–20.
28. Greenwald D, Blum LC 3rd, Adams D, et al. Effective surgical treatment of cubital tunnel syndrome based on provocative clinical testing without electrodiagnostics. Plast Reconstr Surg 2006;117:87e–91e.
29. Martinoli C, Bianchi S, Pugliese F, et al. Sonography of entrapment neuropathies in the upper limb (wrist excluded). J Clin Ultrasound 2004;32:438–50.
30. Vucic S, Cordato DJ, Yiannikas C, et al. Utility of magnetic resonance imaging in diagnosing ulnar neuropathy at the elbow. Clin Neurophysiol 2006;117:590–5.
31. Cobb TK. Endoscopic cubital tunnel release. J Hand Surg Am 2010;35:1690–7.
32. Gervasio O, Zaccone C. Surgical approach to ulnar nerve compression at the elbow caused by the epitrochleoanconeus muscle and a prominent medial head of the triceps. Neurosurgery 2008;62:186–92 [discussion: 192–3].
33. Oertel J, Keiner D, Gaab MR. Endoscopic decompression of the ulnar nerve at the elbow. Neurosurgery 2010;66:817–24 [discussion: 824].
34. Ahcan U, Zorman P. Endoscopic decompression of the ulnar nerve at the elbow. J Hand Surg Am 2007;32:1171–6.
35. Mirza A, Reinhart MK, Bove J, et al. Scope-assisted release of the cubital tunnel. J Hand Surg Am 2011;36:147–51.
36. Bain GI, Bajhau A. Endoscopic release of the ulnar nerve at the elbow using the Agee device: a cadaveric study. Arthroscopy 2005;21:691–5.
37. Dutzmann S, Martin KD, Sobottka S, et al. Open vs retractor-endoscopic in situ decompression of the ulnar nerve in cubital tunnel syndrome: a retrospective cohort study. Neurosurgery 2013;72:605–16 [discussion: 614–6].

Minimal-Incision In Situ Ulnar Nerve Decompression at the Elbow

Joshua M. Adkinson, MD[a], Kevin C. Chung, MD, MS[b,*]

KEYWORDS

• Cubital tunnel syndrome • Ulnar neuropathy • Cubital tunnel release • Minimally invasive surgery • Minimal-incision surgery

KEY POINTS

- Clinical evaluation is paramount in the diagnosis of cubital tunnel syndrome because electrodiagnostic testing often is not sufficiently sensitive to detect changes associated with the syndrome.
- A 1.5- to 3.0-cm longitudinal or transverse skin incision is created at the midpoint between the medial epicondyle and the olecranon, exposing the ulnar nerve; no neurolysis is performed.
- Increasing evidence shows minimally invasive open in situ release to be both safe and effective for the relief of ulnar nerve compression symptoms.

INTRODUCTION

Ulnar nerve entrapment at the elbow is the second most common compression neuropathy in the upper extremity following carpal tunnel syndrome,[1,2] with an estimated prevalence of 1% in the US population.[3] Although earlier descriptions of ulnar neuropathy at the elbow are found in the literature,[4,5] the entity of *cubital tunnel syndrome* was originally proposed by Feindel and Stratford[6,7] in 1958.

Although simple "liberation of the ulnar nerve" was performed as early as 1878,[5] British surgeon Geoffrey Osborne would be the first to gain significant support for simple decompression of the nerve by dividing the eponymous ligament.[2] In his 1957 study,[8] the fibrous connective tissue band spanning the interval between the medial epicondyle and the olecranon was divided. Osborne posited that, in patients with idiopathic ulnar neuropathy at the elbow, simple in situ decompression offered results similar to the more aggressive surgical techniques available.[9]

Trauma and arthritis have both been implicated as causes for ulnar neuropathy. Nevertheless, the most frequent cause of cubital tunnel syndrome remains idiopathic.[2] Multiple potential sites of compression exist along the path of the ulnar nerve. These sites include the arcade of Struthers, the medial intermuscular septum, the anconeus epitrochlearis muscle (if present), the cubital tunnel with the overlying ligament of Osborne, the flexor carpi ulnaris (FCU) muscle, and the flexor-pronator aponeurosis.[10,11] Evidence has also shown that, with elbow flexion and extension, the ulnar nerve lengthens[6,12,13] and is potentially compressed by both dynamic pressure[6,14–17] and shape[6,7,12,18,19] changes within the tunnel.

Supported in part by grants from the National Institute on Aging and National Institute of Arthritis and Musculoskeletal and Skin Diseases (R01 AR062066) and from the National Institute of Arthritis and Musculoskeletal and Skin Diseases (2R01 AR047328-06) and a Midcareer Investigator Award in Patient-Oriented Research (K24 AR053120) (to Dr Kevin C. Chung).
[a] Division of Plastic Surgery, Department of Surgery, Lehigh Valley Health Network, Cedar Crest & I-78, P.O. Box 689, Allentown, PA 18103-4689, USA; [b] Section of Plastic Surgery, University of Michigan Medical School, 2130 Taubman Center, SPC 5340, 1500 East Medical Center Drive, Ann Arbor, MI 48109-5340, USA
* Corresponding author.
E-mail address: kecchung@umich.edu

Hand Clin 30 (2014) 63–70
http://dx.doi.org/10.1016/j.hcl.2013.08.019
0749-0712/14/$ – see front matter

Cubital tunnel syndrome can be treated with a variety of surgical approaches, including simple in situ decompression, epicondylectomy, and various transposition techniques.[2,20,21] Controversy remains, however, regarding the gold standard surgical approach[20] owing to the relatively similar rates of operative successes and failures as well as strong proponents for each technique.[8,22,23]

Since the term *minimally invasive surgery* was first coined by Wickham[24] in 1987, the length of surgical incisions and the extent of soft tissue dissection continue to decrease. Minimally invasive approaches for the treatment of cubital tunnel syndrome are becoming increasingly commonplace as evidence supporting the safety, efficacy, and lower relative morbidity of these procedures accumulates.[25–27] Minimal-incision open in situ cubital tunnel release is discussed further in this article.

Anatomy

Originating from the ventral rami of the C8 and T1 nerve roots, the ulnar nerve is the terminal branch of the medial cord of the brachial plexus. The nerve courses anterior to the medial intermuscular septum, passing through the arcade of Struthers 8 cm proximal to the medial epicondyle. Continuing toward the elbow, the ulnar nerve travels alongside and just posterior to the septum, entering the cubital tunnel between the medial epicondyle and the olecranon. The floor of the cubital tunnel consists of the medial collateral ligament and the elbow joint capsule, and the roof is made of the Osborne ligament as well as the fascia of the FCU. The nerve then travels into the forearm between the humeral and ulnar heads of the FCU and continues in the interval between the FCU and the flexor digitorum profundus muscle bellies[2,11] toward the wrist and hand.

SURGICAL TECHNIQUE

Preoperative Planning

The diagnosis of cubital tunnel syndrome requires a careful examination and history. Symptoms are typically a combination of numbness, weakness, and paresthesias in the ulnar nerve distribution. The initial examination should assess vibratory and light touch sensation in the ulnar distribution. More severe cases can also show abnormal 2-point discrimination, muscle wasting, intrinsic atrophy, and clawing. The examiner may also find positive Wartenberg and Froment signs in more advanced cases.[2,28–36]

There are several provocative tests useful in localizing ulnar neuropathy at the elbow. Although up to 24% of asymptomatic individuals may manifest a positive finding,[37] a Tinel sign is commonly associated with cubital tunnel syndrome and has a 98% negative predictive value.[38,39] Other sensitive and specific clinical findings include the elbow flexion, the cubital tunnel compression test,[40] and the scratch collapse test.[1] This test has recently been described whereby a brief loss of muscle resistance is elicited with skin scratching over the area of nerve compression as patients resist shoulder external rotation.[1] The scratch collapse test has a sensitivity of 69% and an accuracy of 89%.[39] An inching technique, though not mandatory in all patients, may be helpful to determine the exact location of compression.

Clinical evaluation is paramount in the diagnosis of cubital tunnel syndrome because electrodiagnostic testing is not adequately sensitive to detect changes associated with the syndrome.[2,6,28] Nerve studies can be useful in localizing the level of nerve compression while also identifying other concomitant disease processes.[6,28,41] These studies should be considered for all patients because comparative studies can assist in postoperative decision making should the signs and symptoms not improve. If there is concern about a neck, chest, or elbow osseous abnormality, plain radiographs can be helpful.

Conservative treatment (ie, activity modification, padding, splinting) is recommended for those patients with mild symptoms[6,36,42–44]; no benefit has been seen after local steroid injection into the cubital tunnel.[45,46] The goals at this stage of treatment are to decrease both the severity and frequency of symptoms as well as to prevent disease progression. A list of indications and contraindications has been included in **Box 1**. Patients meeting surgical indications and failing nonoperative management are then considered for surgery.

Box 1
Indications and contraindications

Indications

- Ulnar neuropathy at the elbow (mild, moderate, severe)

Contraindications

- Elbow trauma
- Morbid obesity
- Ulnar nerve subluxation at the elbow (preoperatively or intraoperatively)
- Recurrent or persistent postoperative ulnar neuropathy at the elbow

Preparation and Patient Positioning

Anesthesia

Several options exist for anesthesia: general, regional (axillary block), or local infiltration of the operative field (5–10 mL of 1% plain lidocaine or 0.5% bupivacaine into planned incision) with or without sedation.

Position

Patients are in the supine position with the operative arm on an extremity table. The arm is abducted, and the elbow is flexed to 90° and propped on surgical towels.

Surgical approach

- Step 1: The incision is designed as a 1.5- to 3.0-cm longitudinal or transverse skin incision marked at the midpoint between the medial epicondyle and the olecranon (**Fig. 1**).

Some investigators avoid placing the incision directly over the cubital tunnel to prevent a continuous scar extending from the skin to the ulnar nerve.

- Step 2: If a tourniquet is used, the extremity is exsanguinated and the tourniquet is inflated to 250 mm Hg.
- Step 3: The skin incision is made, and the subcutaneous tissue is divided. Extreme care is taken to avoid crossing branches of the medial antebrachial cutaneous nerve (**Fig. 2**). The skin and soft tissues are retracted using Senn retractors.
- Step 4: The fascial layer overlying the nerve is exposed, and the ligament of Osborne is divided using scissors (**Figs. 3** and **4**). Only the superficial surface of the nerve is exposed and no neurolysis is performed, decreasing the likelihood for nerve subluxation. Decompression is carried proximally to the arcade of Struthers and intermuscular septum and distally between the 2 heads of the FCU. Inspection for proximal or distal sites of compression is performed and addressed as necessary. If subluxation is present after in situ release, then transposition is indicated.

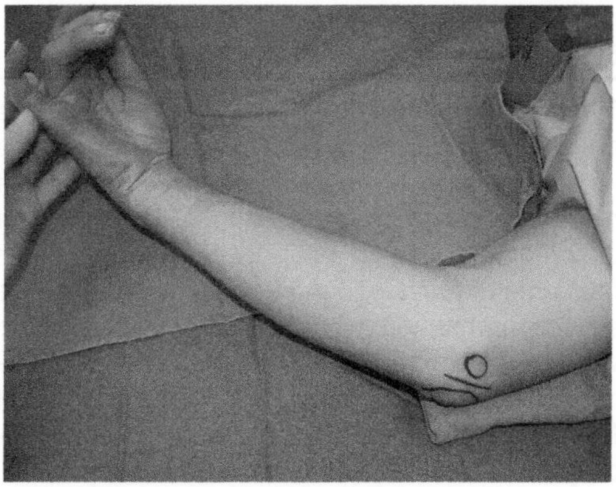

Fig. 1. Preoperative markings for minimal-incision ulnar nerve decompression.

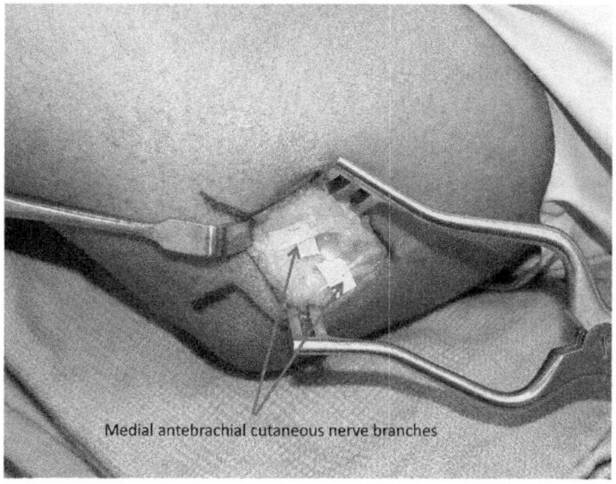

Fig. 2. Care must be taken not to damage the crossing branches of the medial antebrachial cutaneous nerve.

Although Hahn and colleagues[47] noted the equivalent outcomes after minimally invasive medial epicondylectomy with in situ release as compared with anterior subcutaneous transposition, the role of this technical modification is not discussed in this article.

- Step 5: The tourniquet is deflated, and meticulous hemostasis is ensured. The skin is closed in layers with either an interrupted or subcuticular suture in the skin, and a light circumferential dressing is applied without a splint (**Fig. 5**).

Complications

The medial antebrachial cutaneous nerve is at risk with procedures about the medial elbow. The

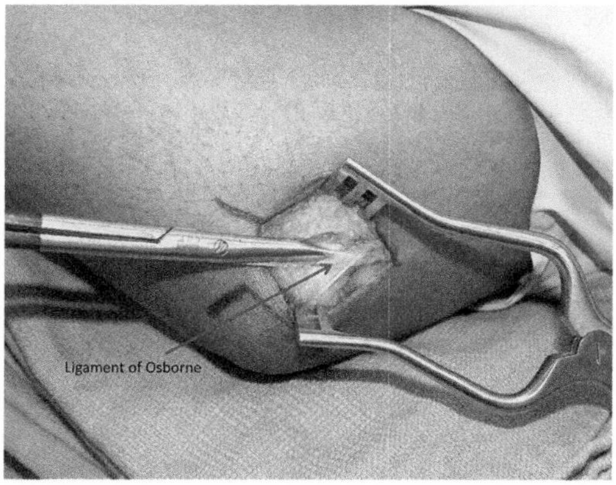

Fig. 3. Ligament of Osborne overlying the ulnar nerve.

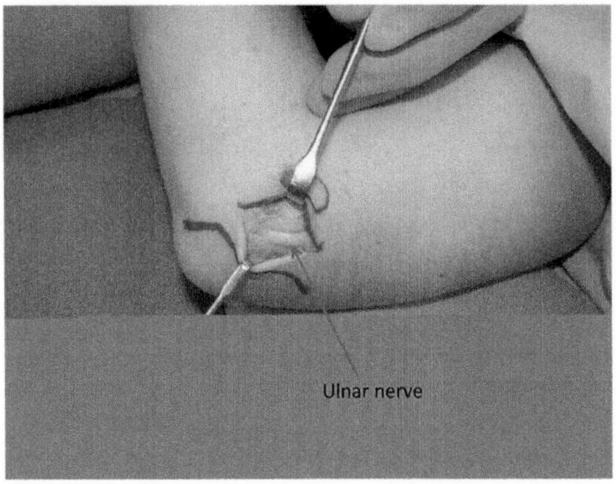

Fig. 4. The ulnar nerve is exposed following incision of the overlying ligament of Osborne and fascial layers.

nerve is known to have branches coursing in an anterior to posterior direction, crossing from 6 cm proximal to 6 cm distal to the medial epicondyle.[48,49] This injury is very poorly tolerated, possibly leading to neuroma, hypesthesia, hyperesthesia, painful scarring,[8,10,49–56] and a possible delay in return to work.[10]

Inadequate release of regional structures is a potential complication of ulnar nerve decompression. No evidence exists regarding the frequency of this complication in patients undergoing minimal-incision in situ release. The most common site of persistent ulnar nerve compression is the origin of the FCU.[56] The intermuscular septum is implicated as a secondary site of compression almost exclusively in those undergoing transposition techniques. The theoretical risks of ulnar nerve compression or kinking at the septum should be minimal with an in situ release.

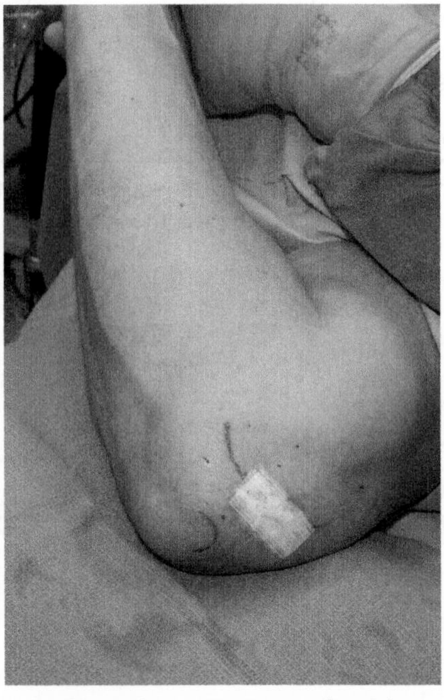

Fig. 5. Postoperative appearance after ulnar nerve decompression.

Iatrogenic injury to the ulnar nerve is also a possible risk, particularly to the motor branches coursing into the FCU.[56] Ulnar nerve instability/subluxation[56–58] and elbow joint instability should be minimal because dissection with an in situ approach is limited. Postoperative scarring leading to perineural fibrosis can cause surgical failure.[58–60]

Postoperative Care

There are no significant postoperative activity restrictions, and the dressing is removed in 2 to 3 days. Scar massage techniques are offered at 3 weeks postoperatively.

OUTCOMES

The fundamental point of contention with regard to surgical management is whether the nerve suffers from compression, traction, or a combination of both[2] and whether both of these factors are clinically significant. The landmark study by Gelberman and colleagues[16] concluded that in situ release failed to change the ulnar nerve intraneural pressure at or 4 cm proximal to the cubital tunnel. This finding resulted in increased disfavor for the in situ approach, particularly among orthopedic surgeons.[2] In contrast, other studies have shown in situ release to be both safe and effective for the relief of ulnar nerve compression symptoms, despite laboratory data showing that the nerve suffers from significant traction with increasing elbow flexion.[22]

Evidence for In Situ Release

Evidence supporting the role of in situ release is abundant (**Table 1**). In addition to the outcomes noted in **Table 1**, excellent to good pain relief has also been demonstrated in 75% to 90% of patients following in situ decompression.[8] The favorable outcomes found in these representative studies, combined with the lower risk for both wound infection and surgical-site tenderness,[22,23,63,65] have generated increased interest for in situ techniques. In situ release also theoretically maintains the intrinsic and extrinsic vascularity of the ulnar nerve.[66] In the setting of an improved complication profile with equivalent

Table 1
Summary of articles comparing in situ release with transposition techniques

	Study Design	Study Population	Outcomes	Complications
Bartels et al,[22] 2005	Prospective comparison of in situ release vs subcutaneous anterior transposition	152 patients followed for 1 y (75 in situ releases, 77 transpositions)	Equivalent	Higher in transposition group
Nabhan et al,[61] 2005	Randomized study of simple decompression vs subcutaneous anterior transposition	66 patients (32 in situ releases, 34 transpositions)	Equivalent	—
Foster & Edshage,[62] 1981	Retrospective review of simple decompression vs subcutaneous anterior transposition	48 cases	Equivalent pain relief improved paresthesia relief and return of intrinsic function with transposition	—
Biggs & Curtis,[63] 2006	Prospective randomized study of in situ release vs submuscular transposition	44 patients (23 in situ releases, 21 transpositions)	Similar rates of improvement (61% in situ vs 67% transposition)	Higher risk for wound complications in transposition group
Caliandro et al,[64] 2011	Cochrane Review comparing simple decompression vs submuscular or subcutaneous transposition	—	Equivalent, even in setting of severe preoperative nerve impairment	Higher risk for infection in transposition group

outcomes, the less invasive, technically simpler option should be selected.

Evidence for Minimal-Incision In Situ Release

Minimally invasive procedures are becoming increasingly popular.[67] This phenomenon is overwhelmingly patient driven; however, benefits of these techniques are apparent. Minimal skin incision cubital tunnel release frequently offers adequate exposure while shortening recuperation time[67] and increasing patient satisfaction.[68] Furthermore, larger incisions (6–10 cm) put the variably located branches of the medial antebrachial cutaneous nerve at risk.

The amount of comparative evidence for the use of minimal-incision cubital tunnel release techniques is growing, and all existing studies show a benefit (**Table 2**). These studies, however, are limited by the lack of control groups, a generally small sample size, and nonstandardized outcomes measures. To address these limitations, the Surgery of the Ulnar Nerve Study Group was formed. The primary objective of this group was to examine outcomes after simple in situ ulnar nerve decompression using a 3-cm incision. The data derived from this collaboration of 5 medical centers were also used to assess for the most responsive presurgical and postsurgical disability instruments. The greatest clinical improvement after in situ decompression was found to occur in the first 6 weeks postoperatively, reaching a plateau by 3 months postoperatively.[73] A review of disability instruments showed that the Michigan Hand Questionnaire (MHQ) and Carpal Tunnel Questionnaire (CTQ) were better able to detect clinically significant postsurgical improvements than the Disabilities of the Arm, Shoulder, and Hand (DASH) Questionnaire.[74] Lastly, despite a small change in MHQ, DASH, and CTQ scores, simple decompression for cubital tunnel syndrome was able to provide objective measures of patient satisfaction.[75]

Table 2
Summary of articles reporting minimal-incision in situ release outcomes

	Study Design	Study Population	Outcomes	Complications
Taniguchi et al,[69] 2002	Prospective study of 1.5- to 2.5-cm incision in situ release	17 patients (18 elbows)	Improved Messina scores, no nerve subluxation	1 hematoma
Cho et al,[70] 2007	Prospective study of <2.0-cm incision in situ release vs traditional in situ release	15 patients (5 treated with minimal incision)	Excellent to good outcomes (Modified Bishop scores)	None, no recurrences or subluxation
Calisaneller et al,[71] 2011	Prospective study of in situ release with two 2-cm incisions (proximal and distal to cubital tunnel)	4 patients	Excellent results (3 of 4 patients), good results (1 of 4) (Wilson and Krout grading system)	None
Jeon et al,[72] 2010	Prospective study of minimal skin incision	66 patients	Satisfactory results in 81% (Messina scores) in patients with McGowan stage I/II disease	2 cases of hematoma

SUMMARY

With initiatives to decrease operative morbidity, complications, and associated costs, minimal-incision techniques have found an expanding role within multiple specialties. Minimal-incision in situ open techniques for ulnar nerve release at the elbow provide adequate exposure and reproducible, satisfactory outcomes. Furthermore, there is no need for endoscopic equipment and the resultant dependence on staff adequately trained to operate and troubleshoot equipment. More robust research with a focus on complications and standard outcome measures will be required to further define the role of minimal-incision techniques. This technical modification, however, augments the increasing armamentarium of the hand surgeon.

REFERENCES

1. Palmer BA, Hughes TB. Cubital tunnel syndrome. J Hand Surg Am 2010;35(1):153–63.
2. Waugh RP, Zlotolow DA. In situ decompression of the ulnar nerve at the cubital tunnel. Hand Clin 2007;23(3):319–27.
3. Song JW, Chung KC, Prosser LA. Treatment of ulnar neuropathy at the elbow: cost-utility analysis. J Hand Surg Am 2012;37(8):1617–29.
4. Earle H. Cases and observations illustrating the influence of the nervous system, in regulating animal heat. Med Chir Trans 1816;7:173–94.
5. Bartels RH. History of the surgical treatment of ulnar nerve compression at the elbow. Neurosurgery 2001;49(2):391–9.
6. Szabo RM, Kwak C. Natural history and conservative management of cubital tunnel syndrome. Hand Clin 2007;23(3):311–8.
7. Feindel W, Stratford J. The role of the cubital tunnel in tardy ulnar palsy. Can J Surg 1958;1(4):287–300.
8. Osborne GV. The surgical treatment of tardy ulnar neuropathy. J Bone Joint Surg Br 1957;39:782.
9. Abuelem T, Ehni BL. Minimalist cubital tunnel treatment. Neurosurgery 2009;65(Suppl 4):A145–9.
10. Bruno W, Tsai T. Minimally invasive release of the cubital tunnel. Operat Tech Plast Reconstr Surg 2002;9:131–7.
11. Polatsch DB, Melone CP Jr, Beldner S, et al. Ulnar nerve anatomy. Hand Clin 2007;23(3):283–9.
12. Apfelberg DB, Larson SJ. Dynamic anatomy of the ulnar nerve at the elbow. Plast Reconstr Surg 1973;51(1):79–81.
13. Contreras MG, Warner MA, Charboneau WJ, et al. Anatomy of the ulnar nerve at the elbow: potential relationship of acute ulnar neuropathy to gender differences. Clin Anat 1998;11(6):372–8.
14. Iba K, Wada T, Aoki M, et al. Intraoperative measurement of pressure adjacent to the ulnar nerve in patients with cubital tunnel syndrome. J Hand Surg Am 2006;31(4):553–8.
15. Werner CO, Ohlin P, Elmqvist D. Pressures recorded in ulnar neuropathy. Acta Orthop Scand 1985;56(5):404–6.

16. Gelberman RH, Yamaguchi K, Hollstien SB, et al. Changes in interstitial pressure and cross-sectional area of the cubital tunnel and of the ulnar nerve with flexion of the elbow: an experimental study in human cadavera. J Bone Joint Surg Am 1998;80(4):492–501.
17. Macnicol MF. Extraneural pressures affecting the ulnar nerve at the elbow. Hand 1982;14(1): 5–11.
18. Vanderpool DW, Chalmers J, Lamb DW, et al. Peripheral compression lesions of the ulnar nerve. J Bone Joint Surg Br 1968;50(4):792–803.
19. Pechan J, Julis I. The pressure measurement in the ulnar nerve: a contribution to the pathophysiology of the cubital tunnel syndrome. J Biomech 1975; 8(1):75–9.
20. Bartels RH, Menovsky T, Van Overbeeke JJ, et al. Surgical management of ulnar nerve compression at the elbow: an analysis of the literature. J Neurosurg 1998;89(5):722–7.
21. Heithoff SJ. Cubital tunnel syndrome does not require transposition of the ulnar nerve. J Hand Surg Am 1999;24(5):898–905.
22. Bartels RH, Verhagen WI, van der Wilt GJ, et al. Prospective randomized controlled study comparing simple decompression versus anterior subcutaneous transposition for idiopathic neuropathy of the ulnar nerve at the elbow: part 1. Neurosurgery 2005;56(3):522–30.
23. Gervasio O, Gambardella G, Zaccone C, et al. Simple decompression versus anterior submuscular transposition of the ulnar nerve in severe cubital tunnel syndrome: a prospective randomized study. Neurosurgery 2005;56(1):108–17.
24. Wickham J. The new surgery. Br Med J (Clin Res Ed) 1987;295(6613):1581–2.
25. Tsai TM, Chen IC, Majd ME, et al. Cubital tunnel release with endoscopic assistance: results of a new technique. J Hand Surg Am 1999;24(1): 21–9.
26. Ahcan U, Zorman PJ. Endoscopic decompression of the ulnar nerve at the elbow. Hand Surg Am 2007;32(8):1171–6.
27. Flores LP. Endoscopically assisted release of the ulnar nerve for cubital tunnel syndrome. Acta Neurochir 2010;152(4):619–25.
28. Mackinnon SE, Novak CB. Compression neuropathies. In: Green DP, Hotchkiss RN, Pederson WC, editors. Green's operative hand surgery. 6th edition. New York: Churchill-Livingstone; 2010. p. 1392–437.
29. McGowen A. The results of transposition of the ulnar nerve for traumatic ulnar neuritis. J Bone Joint Surg Br 1950;32(3):293–301.
30. Posner MA. Compressive neuropathies of the ulnar nerve at the elbow and wrist. Instr Course Lect 2000;49:305–17.
31. Terrono AL, Millender LH. Management of work-related upper-extremity nerve entrapments. Orthop Clin North Am 1996;27(4):783–93.
32. Aoki M, Takasaki H, Muraki T, et al. Strain on the ulnar nerve at the elbow and wrist during throwing motion. J Bone Joint Surg Am 2005; 87(11):2508–14.
33. Burnham RS, Steadward RD. Upper extremity peripheral nerve entrapments among wheelchair athletes: prevalence, location, and risk factors. Arch Phys Med Rehabil 1994;75(5):519–24.
34. Miller RG, Camp PE. Postoperative ulnar neuropathy. JAMA 1979;242(15):1636–9.
35. Cooper D. Nerve injury associated with patient positioning in the operating room. In: Gelberman R, editor. Operative nerve repair and reconstruction, vol. 2, 1st edition. Philadelphia: JB Lippincott; 1991. p. 1231–42.
36. Idler RS. General principles of patient evaluation and nonoperative management of cubital syndrome. Hand Clin 1996;12(2):397–403.
37. Rayan GM, Jensen C, Duke J. Elbow flexion test in the normal population. J Hand Surg 1992; 17(1):86–9.
38. Bozentka DJ. Cubital tunnel syndrome pathophysiology. Clin Orthop Relat Res 1998;351:90–4.
39. Cheng CJ, Mackinnon-Patterson B, Beck JL, et al. Scratch collapse test for evaluation of carpal and cubital tunnel syndrome. J Hand Surg Am 2008; 33(9):1518–24.
40. Novak CB, Lee GW, Mackinnon SE, et al. Provocative testing for cubital tunnel syndrome. J Hand Surg Am 1994;19(5):817–20.
41. Practice parameter for electrodiagnostic studies in ulnar neuropathy at the elbow: summary statement. American Association of Electrodiagnostic Medicine, American Academy of Neurology, American Academy of Physical Medicine and Rehabilitation. Muscle Nerve 1999;22(3):408–11.
42. Dellon AL. Review of treatment results for ulnar nerve entrapment at the elbow. J Hand Surg Am 1989;14(4):688–700.
43. Sunderland S. The intraneural topography of the radial, median and ulnar nerves. Brain 1945;68: 243–99.
44. Blackmore S. Therapist's management of ulnar nerve neuropathy at the elbow. In: Mackin E, editor. Rehabilitation of the hand and upper extremity. St Louis (MO): Mosby; 2002. p. 679–89.
45. McPherson SA, Meals RA. Cubital tunnel syndrome. Orthop Clin North Am 1992;23(1):111–23.
46. Lund AT, Amadio PC. Treatment of cubital tunnel syndrome: perspectives for the therapist. J Hand Ther 2006;19(2):170–8.
47. Hahn SB, Choi YR, Kang HJ, et al. Decompression of the ulnar nerve and minimal medial epicondylectomy with a small incision for cubital tunnel

syndrome: comparison with anterior subcutaneous transposition of the nerve. J Plast Reconstr Aesthet Surg 2010;63(7):1150–5.
48. Lluch AL. Release of ulnar nerve compression at the elbow through a transverse incision. J Shoulder Elbow Surg 1998;7(1):38–42.
49. Lowe JB 3rd, Maggi SP, Mackinnon SE. The position of crossing branches of the medial antebrachial cutaneous nerve during cubital tunnel surgery in humans. Plast Reconstr Surg 2004; 114:692–6.
50. Jackson LC, Hotchkiss RN. Cubital tunnel surgery. Complications and treatment of failures. Hand Clin 1996;12(2):449–56.
51. Masear VR, Meyer RD, Pichora DR. Surgical anatomy of the medial antebrachial cutaneous nerve. J Hand Surg Am 1989;14:267–71.
52. Osterman AL, Davis CA. Subcutaneous transposition of the ulnar nerve for treatment of cubital tunnel syndrome. Hand Clin 1996;12:421–33.
53. Sarris I, Göbel F, Gainer M, et al. Medial brachial and antebrachial cutaneous nerve injuries: effect on outcome in revision cubital tunnel surgery. J Reconstr Microsurg 2002;18:665–70.
54. Tetro AM, Pichora DR. Cubital tunnel syndrome and the painful upper extremity. Hand Clin 1996;12: 665–77.
55. Tomaino MM, Brach PJ, Vansickle DP. The rationale for and efficacy of surgical intervention for electrodiagnostic-negative cubital tunnel syndrome. J Hand Surg Am 2001;26:1077–81.
56. Ruchelsman DE, Lee SK, Posner MA. Failed surgery for ulnar nerve compression at the elbow. Hand Clin 2007;23:359–71.
57. Rogers MR, Bergfield TG, Aulicino PL. The failed ulnar nerve transposition: etiology and treatment. Clin Orthop Relat Res 1991;269:193–200.
58. Vogel RB, Nossaman BC, Rayan GM. Revision anterior submuscular transposition of the ulnar nerve for failed submuscular transposition. Br J Plast Surg 2004;57(4):311–6.
59. Gabel GT, Amadio PC. Reoperation for failed decompression of the ulnar nerve in the region of the elbow. J Bone Joint Surg Am 1990;3(1):213–9.
60. Filippi R, Charalampaki P, Reisch R, et al. Recurrent cubital tunnel syndrome: etiology and treatment. Minim Invasive Neurosurg 2001;44(4): 197–201.
61. Nabhan A, Ahlhelm F, Kelm J, et al. Simple decompression or subcutaneous anterior transposition of the ulnar nerve for cubital tunnel syndrome. J Hand Surg Br 2005;30:521–4.
62. Foster RJ, Edshage S. Factors related to the outcome of surgically managed compressive ulnar neuropathy at the elbow level. J Hand Surg Am 1981;6:181–92.
63. Biggs M, Curtis JA. Randomized, prospective study comparing ulnar neurolysis in situ with submuscular transposition. Neurosurgery 2006;58(2): 296–304.
64. Caliandro P, La Torre G, Padua R, et al. Treatment for ulnar neuropathy at the elbow. Cochrane Database Syst Rev 2011;(2):CD006839.
65. Macadam SA, Gandhi R, Bezuhly M, et al. Simple decompression versus anterior subcutaneous and submuscular transposition of the ulnar nerve for cubital tunnel syndrome: a meta-analysis. J Hand Surg Am 2008;33(8):1314.e1–12.
66. Eversmann WW. Entrapment and compression neuropathies. In: Green DP, editor. Operative hand surgery. 2nd edition. New York: Churchill-Livingstone; 1988. p. 1423–78.
67. Cobb TK. Endoscopic cubital tunnel release. J Hand Surg Am 2010;35(10):1690–7.
68. Ducic I, Endara M, Al-Attar A, et al. Minimally invasive peripheral nerve surgery: a short scar technique. Microsurgery 2010;30:622–6.
69. Taniguchi Y, Takami M, Takami T, et al. Simple decompression with small skin incision for cubital tunnel syndrome. J Hand Surg Br 2002;27(6): 559–62.
70. Cho YJ, Cho SM, Sheen SH, et al. Simple decompression of the ulnar nerve for cubital tunnel syndrome. J Korean Neurosurg Soc 2007;42(5):382–7.
71. Calisaneller T, Ozdemir O, Caner H, et al. Simple decompression of the ulnar nerve at the elbow via proximal and distal mini skin incisions. Turk Neurosurg 2011;21(2):167–71.
72. Jeon IH, Micić I, Lee BW, et al. Simple in situ decompression for idiopathic cubital tunnel syndrome using minimal skin incision. Med Pregl 2010;63(9–10):601–6.
73. Giladi AM, Gaston RG, Haase SC, et al. Trend of recovery after simple decompression for treatment of ulnar neuropathy at the elbow. Plast Recontsr Surg 2013;131(4):563e–73e.
74. Song JW, Waljee JF, Burns PB, et al. An outcome study for ulnar neuropathy at the elbow: a multicenter study by the SUN study group. Neurosurgery 2013;72(6):971–82.
75. Malay S, SUN Study Group, Chung KC. The minimal clinically important difference after simple decompression for ulnar neuropathy at the elbow. J Hand Surg Am 2013;38(4):652–9.

Arthroscopic Excision of Ganglion Cysts

Nicholas A. Bontempo, MD, Arnold-Peter C. Weiss, MD*

KEYWORDS

• Ganglion • Ganglion cyst • Carpal ganglion • Arthroscopic excision

KEY POINTS

- Dorsal carpal ganglions typically arise from the scapholunate ligament.
- Surgical excision, whether open or arthroscopic, should be considered only when the cyst is symptomatic and interferes with daily activities.
- The identification of the stalk arthroscopically has not been shown to correlate with recurrence.
- Recurrence rates following arthroscopic excision of ganglion cysts are as good, if not better, than open excision.
- New techniques are being introduced to help with identification and excision of the ganglion cyst. These techniques include the use of ultrasound and the injection of methylene blue into the cyst.

INTRODUCTION

Ganglions are the most common soft tissue mass of the hand and wrist.[1] Dorsal ganglions are benign soft tissue tumors that arise from the scapholunate ligament.[1] On the surface, these tumors present as variable-sized cysts on the dorsum of the wrist that are soft and transilluminate on physical examination.[1–3] The presence of a ganglion may not cause any symptoms and, thus, are commonly managed with observation. Treatment of the ganglion is indicated once patients experience weakness, pain, difficulty with certain activities, or if the cyst has increased drastically in size.[1–3]

Conservative measures other than observation include aspiration, ganglion puncture, and closed rupture. These measures, however, are associated with recurrence rates reported as high as 78%.[4–6] In order to decrease the rate of recurrence, surgical intervention is recommended. Surgery entails either open or arthroscopic excision of the cyst along with its stalk.

The sac that makes up the dorsal ganglion has a stalk that arises directly from the scapholunate ligament.[1] Surgical excision of the stalk helps to reduce the recurrence of the ganglion after surgery. Regardless of whether the ganglion is removed by open or arthroscopic means, it is necessary to remove the stalk to obtain the lowest rate of recurrence.

Suggested benefits of arthroscopic excision include smaller incisions, less postoperative pain, lower recurrence rates, earlier return to function, and less scarring.[7–12] Recurrence rates following arthroscopic excision of ganglion cysts have been reported from 0% to 17%.[8,9,12–20] Later a technique for arthroscopic excision of dorsal ganglions of the wrist is described.

INDICATIONS/CONTRAINDICATIONS

There is no clear indication in the literature for performing arthroscopic versus open excision of ganglions. Patients who would benefit from arthroscopy are those who require a faster return of function and motion.[13,21] Arthroscopic ganglion excision is only indicated for dorsal carpal ganglions and not for volar carpal ganglions.

Department of Orthopaedics, Warren Alpert Medical School of Brown University, 2 Dudley Street, Suite 200, Providence, RI 02905, USA
* Corresponding author.
E-mail address: apcweiss@brown.edu

Hand Clin 30 (2014) 71–75
http://dx.doi.org/10.1016/j.hcl.2013.08.020

SURGICAL TECHNIQUE

The surgical procedure can be performed in either an ambulatory surgery center or an office operatory suite under general anesthesia, forearm Bier block, or monitored anesthesia care in conjunction with a local anesthetic.

Preparation and Patient Positioning

Patients are placed supine on the operating table, and a forearm or upper arm tourniquet can be applied to the operative extremity. Once anesthesia is induced, an Esmarch bandage is used to exsanguinate the extremity, and the tourniquet is typically raised to 250 mm Hg. Skin can be prepped with any type of surgical scrub, and the extremity is draped in a normal sterile fashion.

Surgical Approach

For an arthroscopic excision of a ganglion cyst, 2 portals are used. First, a 3–4 portal is identified by palpating the Lister tubercle and feeling a soft spot approximately 1 cm distal to it. Second, a 4–5 portal is then identified about 2.0 to 2.5 cm ulnar and slightly proximal to the 3–4 portal. Both of these portals are marked on the skin with a surgical marking pen.

Surgical Procedure

Step 1. Two stab incisions are made at the previously marked 3–4 and 4–5 portals sites. The arthroscope is introduced through the 4–5 portal, and the shaver is inserted into the 3–4 portal.

Step 2. The scapholunate ligament is examined; then, by rotating the arthroscope, the capsule immediately dorsal to the scapholunate ligament is visualized. Frequently, a tear of the dorsal capsule exists.

Step 3. Using the 2.9-mm cutter blade on the shaver, the capsule is debrided around the 3–4 portal entry site (**Fig. 1**). A bluish cyst wall is frequently visualized through the capsular tear or after the initial capsular debridement.

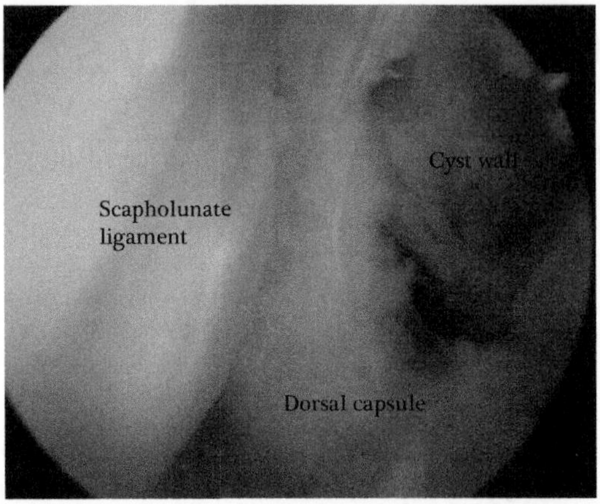

Fig. 1. The dorsal capsule opposite the scapholunate ligament is debrided with the arthroscopic shaver. The cyst wall can frequently be seen through the capsular tear or initial debrided area.

Step 4. The capsular edges are further debrided exposing the extensor carpi radialis brevis (ECRB) tendon initially followed by the extensor pollicis longus (EPL) tendon. The cyst wall is debrided along with the capsule (**Fig. 2**). The surgeon can put external pressure on the cyst pushing it toward the shaver internally to aid in completely debriding the cyst wall and stalk. Frequently, just at the moment of cyst rupture, a transient blurriness occurs from the sudden release of cystic fluid. If the cyst itself is not visualized, debriding the dorsal capsule in the area mentioned should completely decompress the cyst as can be verified by external palpation. One does not need to completely debride the entire cyst wall if a large portion of the wall is removed.

Step 5. Once a wide debridement of the capsule and cyst wall has been performed, the skin can be palpated to demonstrate complete cyst removal (**Fig. 3**).

COMPLICATIONS

Very few complications for this procedure have been described. Laceration of an extensor tendon can occur if, during making the skin portals, the knife goes too deep; care should be undertaken and the blade oriented vertically so that if it

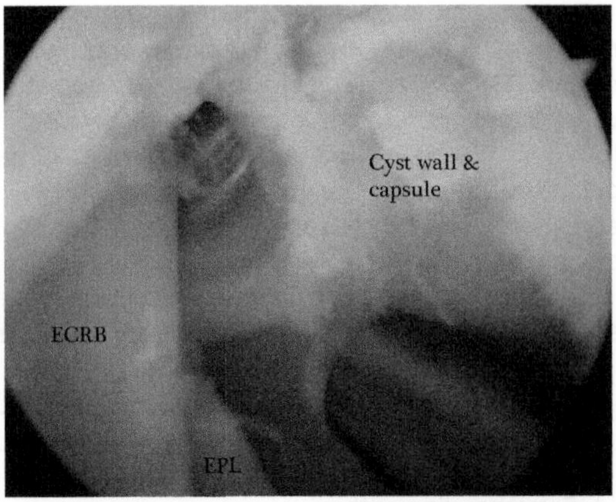

Fig. 2. The shaver is used to further debride the dorsal capsule and cyst wall taking care not to injure the ECRB or EPL tendons.

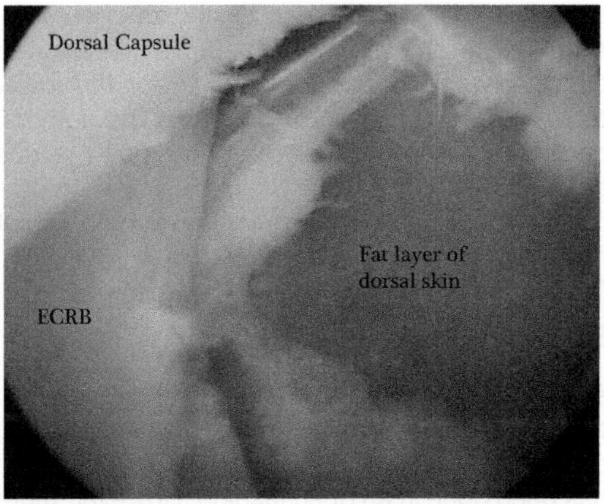

Fig. 3. Following complete debridement of the capsule around the cyst and the cyst wall itself, the dorsal fatty layer of the skin can be visualized and the skin palpated externally to be certain that the cyst has been completely debrided.

does go too deep, then it is in line with the extensor tendons, reducing the risk of complete transection. In addition, care should be taken when debriding the dorsal capsule by identifying the ECRB and EPL tendons and keeping them in view during debridement to avoid any injury to those two tendons.

POSTOPERATIVE CARE

Immediate Postoperative Care

On completion of the surgical procedure, the portal sites are closed with 5–0 nylon sutures, and patients are placed in a volar plaster splint with the wrist in neutral position for 5 to 7 days.

Rehabilitation and Recovery

Patients are seen in the office approximately 5 to 7 days after the surgery, at which time the dressing and splint are taken down and the incisions are inspected. Sutures are typically removed at the first postoperative visit. Patients are then allowed to begin active and passive wrist motion, and no further splinting is used. Additionally, the patients have no restrictions in terms of activity or weight lifting. The patients are seen back at 4 to 8 weeks postoperatively for a repeat clinical evaluation.

CLINICAL RESULTS

The primary outcome of interest in the literature after arthroscopic ganglion excision is recurrence rates. These rates have been reported from 0% to 17% (**Table 1**).[8,9,12–20] Osterman and Raphael[9] conducted a study in which 18 patients underwent arthroscopic excision of dorsal ganglions. In their study, the stalk could be identified in 61% of the cases, and the reported number of recurrences at an average of 16 months was 0. In a slightly larger study of 30 patients, Luchetti and colleagues[8] reported the ability to identify the stalk in 79% of cases, and 2 of the patients had a recurrence at the final follow-up. Edwards and Johansen[15] reported a 0% recurrence in their study of 45 patients and were able to identify the stalk in only 16% of the cases.

Three studies were conducted from 2004 to 2006 by Mathoulin and colleagues,[16] Rizzo and colleagues,[14] and Rocchi and colleagues[18] that reported recurrence rates of dorsal ganglion cysts

Table 1
Recurrence rates of following arthroscopic excision of dorsal ganglions and the rates of intra-operative stalk identification

Author/Year Published	Number of Cases	Number of Recurrences	Recurrence Rate (%)	Ability to Identify Stalk (%)
Osterman & Raphael,[9] 1995	18	0	0	61.0
Luchetti et al,[8] 2000	30	2	6.7	79.0
Mathoulin et al,[16] 2004	96	4	4.2	N/A
Rizzo et al,[14] 2004	41	2	4.9	N/A
Rocchi et al,[18] 2006	30	2	6.7	N/A
Kang et al,[12] 2008	28	3	11.0	100
Edwards & Johansen,[15] 2009	45	0	0	16.0
Gallego et al,[13] 2010	114	14	12.3	100
Chen et al,[17] 2010	15	1	6.7	10.0
Yamamoto et al,[19] 2012	22	2	9.0	18.2
Aslani et al,[20] 2012	52	9	17.3	100

Abbreviation: N/A, Not Available.

following arthroscopic excision of 4.2%, 4.9%, and 6.7%, respectively. None of the 3 studies commented on the ability to identify the stalk arthroscopically.

Two years later, Kang and colleagues[12] conducted a prospective study comparing arthroscopic versus open excision of dorsal ganglion cysts. Forty-one patients underwent arthroscopic excision, and 31 patients underwent open excision. At the second postoperative visit (4–8 weeks postoperative) 1 of the 41 patients who underwent arthroscopic excision versus 0 of the 31 patients who underwent open excision developed a recurrence. At the final follow-up, however, several patients were lost to follow-up; 3 of the remaining 28 patients (11%) in the arthroscopic group and 2 of the remaining 23 patients (9%) had developed a recurrence ($P = .809$). In addition, the investigators were able to identify the stalk in 100% of the cases.

In the largest study to date, Gallego and Mathoulin[13] reported on 114 cases in which arthroscopic excision of ganglion cysts was performed with 2-year follow-up data. In their study, 14 patients (12.3%) had a recurrence at the final follow-up, and the stalk was identified in 100% of the cases. That same year, Chen and colleagues[17] presented 15 cases that had been done arthroscopically, with only 1 recurrence (6.7%) at the 15-month follow-up.

Most recently, 2 studies have been published in 2012 looking at outcomes following arthroscopic excision of ganglion cysts.[19,20] Aslani and colleagues[20] reported on 15 patients, of which 9 (17.3%) developed a recurrence with a range of follow-up of 24 to 71 months. Yamamoto and colleagues[19] recently described a technique by which ultrasound was used as a supplemental tool during arthroscopy to identify the ganglion stalk, the shaver tip, and adjacent neurovascular structures. In their study of 22 patients, there were 2 recurrences (9%); the cyst stalk was only able to be identified 18.2% of the time. Whether the stalk can be identified intraoperatively varies among the reports in the literature, and the clinical importance remains unclear. In 2011, Lee and colleagues[22] described a technique by which methylene blue was injected into the cyst in order to help identify the stalk within the joint.

Most studies have not shown a statistically improved reduction in postoperative pain or functional recovery following an arthroscopic ganglionectomy. Patients, especially women who wear bracelets, appreciate the lack of a larger scar on the dorsal wrist. The internal work involved in removing the cyst is not substantially different from an open excision, so the pain and discomfort expected should be similar. Lastly, an open excision may remove more neutrally innervated capsule, which might compensate for the lower trauma of an arthroscopic excision. The authors' decision tree on whether to use an open versus arthroscopic approach is by explaining both procedures to patients and letting them decide. About half pick each approach.

SUMMARY

Arthroscopy is an advancing field in orthopedics, the applications of which have been expanding over time. Traditionally, excision of ganglion cysts has been done in an open fashion. However, more recently, studies show outcomes following arthroscopic excision to be as good as open excision. Cosmetically, the incisions are smaller and heal faster following arthroscopy. In addition, there is the suggested benefit that patients will regain function and return to work faster following arthroscopic excision. More prospective studies comparing open and arthroscopic excision of ganglion cysts need to be done in order to delineate if there is a true functional benefit.

REFERENCES

1. Athanasian E. Bone and soft tissue tumors. In: Wolfe S, Pederson WC, Kozin S, editors. Green's operative hand surgery. New York: Churchill Livingstone; 2011. p. 2150–95.
2. Thornburg LE. Ganglions of the hand and wrist. J Am Acad Orthop Surg 1999;7(4):231–8.
3. Angelides AC, Wallace PF. The dorsal ganglion of the wrist: its pathogenesis, gross and microscopic anatomy, and surgical treatment. J Hand Surg 1976;1(3):228–35.
4. Richman JA, Gelberman RH, Engber WD, et al. Ganglions of the wrist and digits: results of treatment by aspiration and cyst wall puncture. J Hand Surg 1987;12(6):1041–3.
5. Stephen AB, Lyons AR, Davis TR. A prospective study of two conservative treatments for ganglia of the wrist. J Hand Surg Br 1999;24(1):104–5.
6. Zubowicz VN, Ishii CH. Management of ganglion cysts of the hand by simple aspiration. J Hand Surg 1987;12(4):618–20.
7. Geissler WB, Freeland AE, Weiss AP, et al. Techniques of wrist arthroscopy. Instr Course Lect 2000;49:225–37.
8. Luchetti R, Badia A, Alfarano M, et al. Arthroscopic resection of dorsal wrist ganglia and treatment of recurrences. J Hand Surg Br 2000;25(1):38–40.
9. Osterman AL, Raphael J. Arthroscopic resection of dorsal ganglion of the wrist. Hand Clin 1995;11(1): 7–12.

10. Gupta R, Bozentka DJ, Osterman AL. Wrist arthroscopy: principles and clinical applications. J Am Acad Orthop Surg 2001;9(3):200–9.
11. Bienz T, Raphael JS. Arthroscopic resection of the dorsal ganglia of the wrist. Hand Clin 1999;15(3):429–34.
12. Kang L, Akelman E, Weiss AP. Arthroscopic versus open dorsal ganglion excision: a prospective, randomized comparison of rates of recurrence and of residual pain. J Hand Surg 2008;33(4):471–5.
13. Gallego S, Mathoulin C. Arthroscopic resection of dorsal wrist ganglia: 114 cases with minimum follow-up of 2 years. Arthroscopy 2010;26(12):1675–82.
14. Rizzo M, Berger RA, Steinmann SP, et al. Arthroscopic resection in the management of dorsal wrist ganglions: results with a minimum 2-year follow-up period. J Hand Surg 2004;29(1):59–62.
15. Edwards SG, Johansen JA. Prospective outcomes and associations of wrist ganglion cysts resected arthroscopically. J Hand Surg 2009;34(3):395–400.
16. Mathoulin C, Hoyos A, Pelaez J. Arthroscopic resection of wrist ganglia. Hand Surg 2004;9(2):159–64.
17. Chen AC, Lee WC, Hsu KY, et al. Arthroscopic ganglionectomy through an intrafocal cystic portal for wrist ganglia. Arthroscopy 2010;26(5):617–22.
18. Rocchi L, Canal A, Pelaez J, et al. Results and complications in dorsal and volar wrist ganglia arthroscopic resection. Hand Surg 2006;11(1–2):21–6.
19. Yamamoto M, Kurimoto S, Okui N, et al. Sonography-guided arthroscopy for wrist ganglion. J Hand Surg 2012;37(7):1411–5.
20. Aslani H, Najafi A, Zaaferani Z. Prospective outcomes of arthroscopic treatment of dorsal wrist ganglia. Orthopedics 2012;35(3):e365–70.
21. Geissler WB. Arthroscopic excision of dorsal wrist ganglia. Techn Hand Up Extrem Surg 1998;2(3):196–201.
22. Lee BJ, Sawyer GA, Dasilva MF. Methylene blue-enhanced arthroscopic resection of dorsal wrist ganglions. Techn Hand Up Extrem Surg 2011;15(4):243–6.

Minimally Invasive Approaches to Ulnar-Sided Wrist Disorders

Joseph M. Pirolo, MD, Jeffrey Yao, MD*

KEYWORDS

• Ulnar sided • Wrist pain • Triangular fibrocartilage complex • Ulnocarpal impaction
• Lunotriquetral ligament • Hamate arthrosis

KEY POINTS

- The cause of ulnar-sided wrist pain is often multifactorial.
- A thorough understanding of the anatomy, examination, and radiographic evaluation is essential when treating ulnar-sided wrist pain.
- Arthroscopy is particularly well suited to both directly visualize and treat multiple causes of ulnar sided wrist pain simultaneously.
- Arthroscopic treatment modalities for degenerative conditions such as ulnocarpal impaction and hamate arthrosis include debridement, chondroplasty, microfracture and resection.
- Low grade injury to the lunotriquetral interosseous ligament and the triangular fibrocartilage complex are often amenable to simple debridement and/or thermal shrinkage, while higher grade injuries necessitate repair.

INTRODUCTION: NATURE OF THE PROBLEM

Ulnar-sided wrist pain is a common cause of disability and has long been a diagnostic and therapeutic dilemma for practitioners, earning its titles such as the *black box* and the *low back pain of the wrist*. A thorough understanding of the anatomy, injury mechanisms, and typical clinical presentation will help establish a focused differential diagnosis. The purpose of this article is to review the evaluation and arthroscopic treatment options for the common causes of ulnar-sided wrist pain, including triangular fibrocartilage complex (TFCC) lesions, ulnocarpal impaction syndrome (UIS), lunotriquetral ligament (LTIL) tears, and hamate arthrosis.

THE TFCC

The TFCC is an important stabilizer of the wrist, and multiple studies have clarified its role in stabilization and load transmission.[1–5] TFCC tears are a major source of ulnar-sided wrist pain, and these injuries may result in significant patient disability.[6]

Patients with TFCC injuries present with mechanical wrist pain, which is exacerbated by activities that load the ulnar wrist. Acute injuries to the TFCC often occur in the setting of a fall with axial load to an extended wrist and extremes of forearm rotation. TFCC tears may be associated with pain, swelling, weakness, and a sense of instability.

The physical examination typically reveals a positive fovea sign that is tender to deep palpation in the soft spot between the ulnar styloid and flexor carpi ulnaris with the wrist in neutral rotation.[7] Ulnocarpal stress testing is performed by applying an axial load to the maximally ulnar-deviated wrist and bringing it through pronation and supination. It is a sensitive but nonspecific test for ulnar-sided pathologic conditions including TFCC tears.[8]

Imaging is an important tool in the workup of TFCC injuries. Plain radiographs are useful to assess for acute or prior trauma, ulnar variance, arthritis, and malalignment. Magnetic resonance

Department of Orthopaedic Surgery, Robert A. Chase Hand and Upper Limb Center, Stanford University Medical Center, 450 Broadway Street, M/C 6342, Redwood City, CA 94063, USA
* Corresponding author.
E-mail address: jyao@stanford.edu

Hand Clin 30 (2014) 77–89
http://dx.doi.org/10.1016/j.hcl.2013.09.001
0749-0712/14/$ – see front matter

imaging (MRI) with a 3.0-T magnet has been shown to have 97% accuracy in detection and 92% accuracy in localization for TFCC tears, although this depends on having an experienced musculoskeletal radiologist.[9,10]

Tears are categorized to help in treatment planning. Tears are divided into traumatic (type 1) or degenerative (type 2) according to the Palmer classification system.[11,12] Type 1A tears are generally not destabilizing to the distal radioulnar joint (DRUJ), whereas type 1B, 1C, and 1D lesions may destabilize the DRUJ and, thus, warrant a thorough evaluation for instability.[5,13] Although not formally included in the Palmer criteria, longitudinal split tears of the ulnotriquetral ligament may be grouped into the 1C category and are a source of chronic ulnar-sided pain.

Indications/Contraindications

Treatment of traumatic TFCC injuries typically begins with nonoperative measures, including immobilization, activity modification, and steroid injections. Park and colleagues[14] found that 57% of patients with TFCC injuries achieved resolution of symptoms following 4 weeks of immobilization.

For those patients who fail conservative treatment, arthroscopic debridement and possible repair are excellent treatment options.

Although not a strict contraindication, ulnar positive variance increases failure rates for both debridement and repair of the TFCC.[15–17] Increased failure rates for surgical repair of peripheral tears have also been reported in patients with advanced age, decreased supination, and loss of grip strength.[18]

Surgical Technique

Preoperative planning

Most patients must have failed conservative measures before surgery is considered. Preoperative MRI assists the surgeon in anticipating the intraoperative findings.

Preparation and patient positioning

A standard wrist arthroscopy tower is used with 10-12 lbs (4.5-5.4 kgs) of longitudinal traction placed on the index and long fingers to distract the radiocarpal joint.

Surgical approach

The standard 3–4, 4–5, and 6R portals are used for diagnostic arthroscopy.

Step 1: The stability of the TFCC should be determined using a probe to check the trampoline effect and by hooking the TFCC at the prestyloid recess.

Step 2: The type of tear is determined because the treatment algorithms vary by type.

Step 3: Treatment

Central (Palmer 1A tear) These tears do not heal because of a lack of vascularity and are, thus, treated with simple debridement to a stable edge using a 3.5-mm full-radius motorized shaver and/or a radiofrequency probe (**Fig. 1**A, B).[19] If a radiofrequency probe is used, it is important to apply it intermittently and to have an adequate outflow portal to avoid overheating. Degenerative tears in the setting of a stable DRUJ are also treated with simple debridement to a stable edge.

Peripheral (Palmer 1B) These tears are debrided with a shaver to stimulate angiogenesis at the repair site (**Fig. 2**A). Although multiple repair options are described, the authors prefer to use a FasT-Fix method.[20–27] With the arthroscope in the 6R portal, the curved FasT-Fix (Smith & Nephew Endoscopy, Andover, MA) is inserted through the 3–4 portal with the assistance of the split cannula (see **Fig. 2**B). The first polylactic

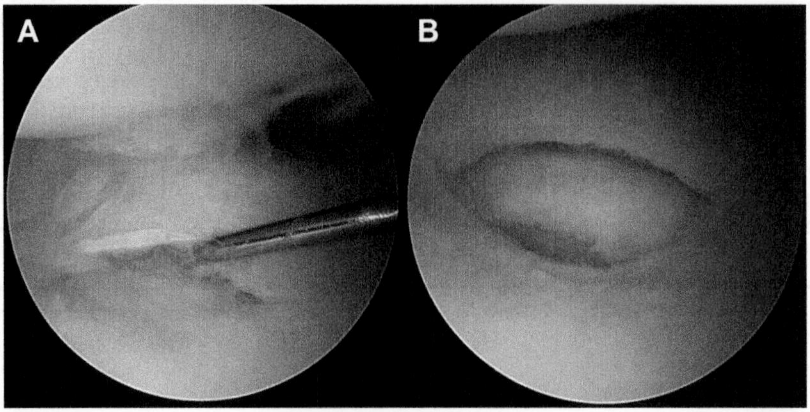

Fig. 1. Central tear is hooked to assess stability (*A*) and then debrided back to a stable edge (*B*).

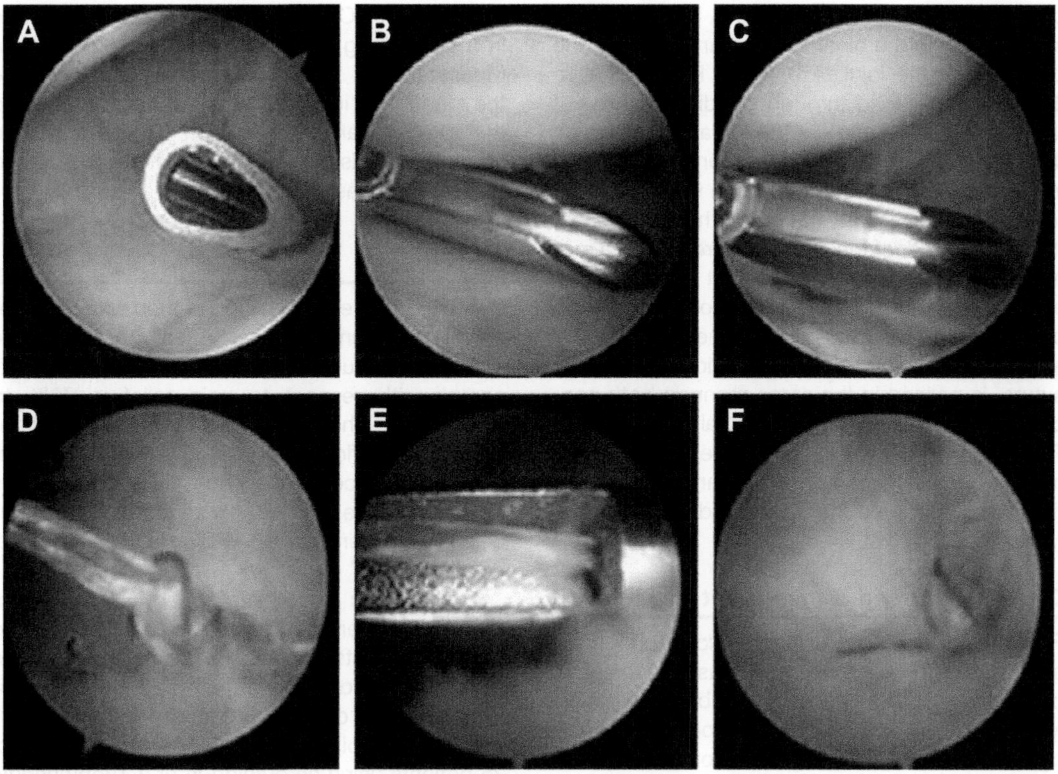

Fig. 2. A 3.5-mm motorized shaver is used to debride the peripheral tear (*A*). The curved FasT-Fix (Smith & Nephew Endoscopy, Andover, MA) is inserted through the 3–4 portal (*B*), then through the TFCC radial to the tear, and then the ulnar capsule (*C*). Deployment of the second block forms a vertical mattress configuration (*D*), which is then cut using an arthroscopic knot cutter (*E, F*).

acid (PLLA) block is inserted radial to the tear, then advanced through the articular disk of the TFCC, and further advanced through the ulnar capsule. The needle introducer is then drawn back, releasing the block from the introducer and depositing the block on the outside of the ulnar wrist capsule. The trigger on the needle introducer is used to advance the second block into the deployment position. The second block is advanced and deposited in the same fashion, ulnar to the tear (approximately 3 mm from the first block), forming a vertical mattress configuration (see **Fig. 2**C). The needle introducer is removed from the joint, leaving the pretied suture (see **Fig. 2**D). The suture is tightened, and the knot is cut by the knot pusher/cutter (see **Fig. 2**E). Once the repair is completed, adequate restoration of the trampoline effect should be achieved (see **Fig. 2**F). A second implant, if necessary, is placed adjacent (typically dorsal) to the initial implant. Stability of the DRUJ is confirmed at this point.

The ulnar extrinsic ligaments should also be evaluated. If a longitudinal split tear is encountered, an outside-in repair is performed as described by Tay and colleagues.[28] A 1-cm longitudinal incision is made just anterior to the extensor carpi ulnaris tendon starting distal to the ulnar styloid process, protecting the dorsal sensory branch of the ulnar nerve and basilic vein. This incision is then used to pass the suture using meniscal needles from outside to inside and then tied down to close the split tear.

Radial-sided (Palmer 1D) avulsions These avulsions are first debrided back to a stable margin. Although multiple techniques have been reported for repair, the authors prefer simple debridement because of the lack of vascularity of the radial aspect of the TFCC.[19,29] However, if DRUJ instability is present because of the radial avulsion, repair may be indicated. The authors prefer a modified technique described by Sagerman and Short.[30] Debridement is performed to a bleeding bony surface at the insertion site on the sigmoid notch of the radius. A 1.5-cm longitudinal incision is made over the ulnar wrist to protect the dorsal sensory branch of the ulnar nerve and over the radial wrist proximal to the styloid to protect the superficial radial nerve. The arthroscope is placed in the 3–4 portal, and a probe is placed in the 6R portal and used as a retractor. A cannula is inserted through the ulnar incision and through the capsule into the joint. A 0.062-in Kirschner wire (k-wire) is advanced through the distal aspect of the sigmoid notch and out the radial wrist incision (**Fig. 3**A). The k-wire is withdrawn and readvanced in the same manner starting 2 mm volar or dorsal to the first pass. With the 2 drill holes in place, the radial border of the TFCC is pierced with a meniscal needle in line with the first drill hole and advanced under arthroscopic vision through the drill hole (see **Fig. 3**B). A second meniscal needle, attached to the first by a 2-0 Polydioxanone (PDS) suture, is passed in the same manner; both needles are retrieved through the radial wrist incision. This action pulls the PDS suture in horizontal mattress fashion, closing the tear. The knot is tied over a bone bridge on the radial side of the radius (see **Fig. 3**C).

Complications and Management

Failure rates for both arthroscopic debridement and repair of TFCC tears are increased in the ulnar positive wrist. Failure has been attributed to underlying degenerative TFCC and ulnocarpal pathology.[15–17] Ulnar shortening osteotomy remains a viable treatment option for those with persistent pain, even in the absence of ulnar positive variance.[17,31] Other complications, such as sensory nerve injury, suture granulomas, and extensor carpi ulnaris tendonitis, are rare but have been reported.[32–34]

Postoperative Care

If TFCC debridement alone is performed, patients are placed in a well-padded volar short arm splint for 2 weeks. If a peripheral repair is performed, the authors' protocol is for placement in a well-molded sugar tong splint with the forearm in neutral rotation for 2 weeks followed by placement of a short arm cast for an additional 4 weeks. This accelerated rehabilitation is afforded by the increased biomechanical strength of the FasT-Fix repair.[35]

If a radial TFCC repair is performed, patients are in a sugar tong splint for 2 weeks followed by a Muenster cast for an additional 4 weeks. Once the period of immobilization is complete, hand therapy for range of motion and progressive strengthening is begun. Full activity is anticipated at 3 to 6 months.[21]

Outcomes

Central TFCC tears are often treated with debridement alone, and success rates are good. The most recent studies report good or excellent outcomes with respect to pain relief in 73% to 87%.[15,36–40] The failure rates of TFCC debridement are significantly higher in patients with ulnar positive variance, ranging from 13% to 60%. This failure to relieve pain is likely secondary to the underlying degenerative TFCC and ulnocarpal pathology.[15–17]

Arthroscopic repairs of Palmer 1B TFCC tears have been generally promising, with good to excellent results reported in a range of 61% to 91% based mostly on patient satisfaction questionnaires and clinical outcome measures.[24,41–43] Estrella and colleagues[24] reported on a series of 35 patients using an outside-in or a Tuohy needle technique and found 74% good to excellent results at an average of 39 months using the modified Mayo wrist score, although this cohort included some Palmer 1C and 1D tears. Corso and colleagues[43] used an outside-in technique in 44 patients and reported good to excellent results in 91% based on preoperative and postoperative modified Mayo wrist scores. Yao and Lee[21] performed arthroscopic FasT-Fix repair of patients with 1B tears, with 11 of 12 patients reporting excellent results based on the Quick Disabilities of the Arm, Shoulder, and Hand (QuickDASH) and Patient-Rated Wrist Evaluation questionnaires. More recently, Wolf and colleagues[44] compared short and midterm results in a group of 40 patients, finding further improvement over time in pain, wrist scores, grip strength, and

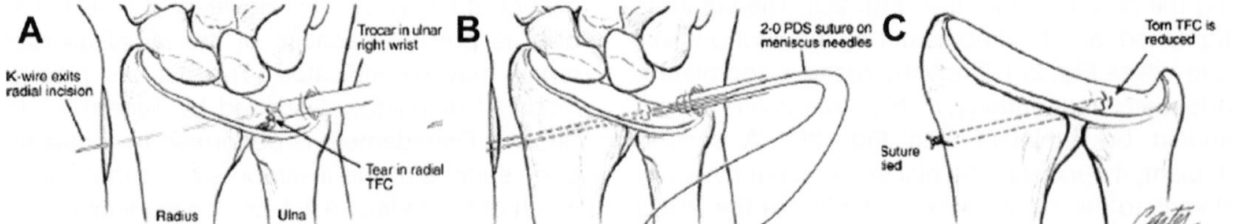

Fig. 3. A 0.062-in k-wire is advanced through the distal aspect of the sigmoid notch and out the radial wrist incision (*A*). The radial border of the TFCC is pierced with a meniscal needle in line with the first drill hole and advanced under arthroscopic vision through the drill hole (*B*). The Polydioxanone (PDS) suture is placed in a horizontal mattress fashion, closing the tear. The knot is tied over a bone bridge on the radial side of the radius (*C*).

motion. In addition to capsular-based repairs, there have been multiple descriptions of direct foveal repairs, which have also shown good success.[32,33,45,46] There is new evidence that Palmer 1B tears may be adequately treated with debridement alone, with Cardenas-Montemayor and colleagues[47] reporting good or excellent results in 87% of patients in their 31 patient series.

Tay and colleagues[28] described an outside-in technique for repair of ulnar extrinsic longitudinal split-tears in a series of 36 patients and reported 89% patient satisfaction and 90% of the patients having no limitations of activity.

Radial sided (Palmer 1D) lesions are technically challenging to repair and are thought to have lower potential for healing secondary to poor vascularity.[19,29] Saegerman described an outside-in transosseous technique combined with pinning of the distal radioulnar joint and noted 67% good or excellent clinical results in a series of 14 patients.[30] Trumble and colleagues[48] described an inside-out transosseous suture technique and reported complete pain relief in 13 of 15 patients. More recently, Tang and colleagues[34] described a technique using a meniscal–double barrel cannula more commonly used in knee arthroscopy. In their review of 11 patients, they reported 50% excellent or good results and 50% fair results.

Summary

For Palmer 1A TFCC lesions, arthroscopic debridement alone is generally a successful procedure. Palmer 1B lesions may be amenable to simple debridement; however, both capsular and direct foveal repairs are generally recommended. Positive ulnar variance may lower the likelihood of success for arthroscopic treatment of TFCC pathology. Ulnar shortening osteotomy remains a successful secondary procedure for persistent pain following debridement or repair of the TFCC. The authors recommend simple debridement of Palmer 1C and 1D lesions except in cases when the DRUJ is unstable and repair may be indicated.

ULNAR IMPACTION SYNDROME AND ULNOCARPAL CHONDROMALACIA

UIS occurs when the TFCC is pathologically compressed in the distal ulnocarpal joint. Ulnar impaction leads to both traumatic and degenerative TFCC tears, ulnocarpal chondromalacia, and injuries to the lunotriquetral ligament. When compared with the ulnar-neutral wrist, as little as a 2-mm increase in ulnar variance will nearly double the force borne by the ulnocarpal joint, whereas a 2-mm decrease will reduce it to a 4% share of the total force transmitted across the wrist.[4]

On clinical examination, tenderness in the ulnocarpal fovea or in the ulnocarpal space dorsally is common. An ulnar impaction test is performed by bringing the wrist forcefully into ulnar deviation, which will reproduce symptoms. Imaging starts with plain radiographs to be assessed for positive ulnar variance and subchondral lucency in the proximal aspects of the lunate and triquetrum. Advanced imaging, including standard MRI or MR arthrography, may be used to confirm a signal change in the central avascular zone of the TFCC, the proximal lunate, triquetrum, and distal ulna.

Treatment of both traumatic and degenerative TFCC pathology may be complicated by the presence of ulnocarpal chondral lesions. Although ulnar positive variance is known to decrease the likelihood of success when treating TFCC tears, it is unknown how chondral lesions within the lunate and triquetrum may affect outcome. Furthermore, there are no descriptions in the literature on how to address these chondral defects during surgery. The authors discuss their practice of chondroplasty and microfracture in this section. This procedure, although common in the knee, ankle, and hip, has yet to be described in the wrist.

Indications/Contraindications

Arthroscopic management for UIS includes the wafer procedure.[16,49–53] Surgical indications for arthroscopic wafer resection (AWR) include ulnar-sided wrist pain with activities, ulnar positive variance, and Palmer 1A, 2C, 2D, or 2E TFCC lesions that fail to respond to conservative treatment. Wafer resection may be preferred over ulnar shortening osteotomy (USO) in patients with concerns for nonunion (comorbidities such as diabetes mellitus, smoking, chronic immunosuppression) or hardware irritation (thinner patients). Contraindications for AWR include ulnar positive variance greater than 5 mm (such as in the setting of distal radius fractures) and the presence of a peripheral TFCC tear.

Surgical Approach

Step 1: The standard distraction tower and arthroscope are used. The 3–4 and 6R portals are used for diagnostic arthroscopy to confirm the diagnosis of ulnocarpal impaction.

Step 2: A suction punch and shaver are alternately placed through the 4–5 portal to debride the TFCC tear to a stable margin and to debride inflamed synovium, border flaps, and any irregularities of the lunotriquetral ligament. Overzealous debridement of the TFCC must be avoided in order to avoid destabilizing the DRUJ. Biomechanical studies have shown that up to 80% of the central articular disk may be resected before causing instability.[54,55]

Step 3: The ulnar head may be visualized through the debrided central TFCC perforation (**Fig. 4**A). A 3.5-mm motorized burr is used to resect the remaining articular cartilage and 2 to 4 mm of subchondral bone from the distal ulna (see **Fig. 4**B). The burr may also be placed beneath the TFCC through the DRUJ portal.[52]

Step 4: The articular surfaces of the lunate and triquetrum are also inspected, and loose cartilage flaps are resected with a motorized shaver to a stable edge to prevent propagation. Following chondroplasty, focal chondral defects are treated with microfracture using an angled awl from an ankle microfracture set. The awl is impacted to penetrate the subchondral bone (**Fig. 5**A). The tourniquet is temporarily released to ensure adequate cortical penetration and medullary bleeding that will allow for clot formation at the chondral defect (see **Fig. 5**B).

Laser AWR has also been described.[53] An assistant must pronate and supinate the forearm through a full arc of motion to ensure circumferential resection of the radial surface of the ulnar head. Fluoroscopy is used to confirm adequate resection with a goal of 2 to 3 mm of ulnar negative variance (see **Fig. 4**C).

Complications

Although rare, minor complications, including postoperative tendonitis, ulnocarpal scar formation, portal site erythema, and dorsal wrist ganglions, have been reported.[16,53] Loss of rotation has also been reported when combined with TFCC debridement.[56] Pitfalls include inadequate resection of the ulnar head and overzealous debridement of the TFCC leading to instability.

Postoperative Care

Following AWR, pronation and supination are allowed in the volar splint immediately and the splint is discontinued after 1 week. Range-of-motion exercises are initiated with hand therapy starting 10 days following surgery. The wrist should be protected in a cock-up wrist brace during therapy. Gradual progression of the rehabilitation regimen is dictated by patient comfort, and grip strengthening is started at approximately 4 weeks. Patients with a microfracture are immobilized for 6 weeks to allow for the attachment and maturation of the clot into fibrocartilage. Motion before this may lead to shearing and destabilization of the clot from the underlying subchondral bone.

Outcomes

Studies evaluating the results of AWR for the treatment of UIS have shown similar to favorable results compared with USO.[16,53,56–60] In a comparison of arthroscopic TFCC debridement followed by either AWR or USO, Bernstein and colleagues[16] found AWR to have equivalent results with fewer complications and fewer secondary procedures.[16] Vandenberghe and colleagues[60] compared AWR versus USO and found no statistical differences in DASH scores, Visual Analog Scores (VAS), and return to work. Tomaino and Weisner[56] reported 12 out of 12 were either very satisfied or satisfied, with 11 out of 12 patients back to work by 8 weeks.[56] Nagle and Bernstein[53] reported good or excellent results in 9 out of 11 patients treated with laser-assisted AWR. Meftah and colleagues[58] reported 22 out of 26 patients had either good or excellent pain relief and found a significant correlation between the presence of MRI findings, such as cystic changes, edema, or sclerosis, and postoperative pain relief. They also report a correlation between prior distal radius fracture and poor outcomes. Although there are no descriptions of

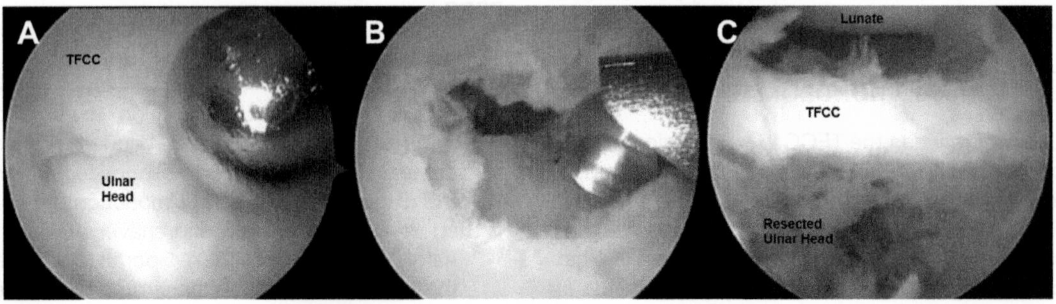

Fig. 4. Following debridement of the central TFCC tear using a suction punch and shaver, the ulnar head is identified (*A*). A 3.5-mm motorized burr is used to resect cartilage and subchondral bone to a goal of 2- to 3-mm ulnar negative variance (*B, C*).

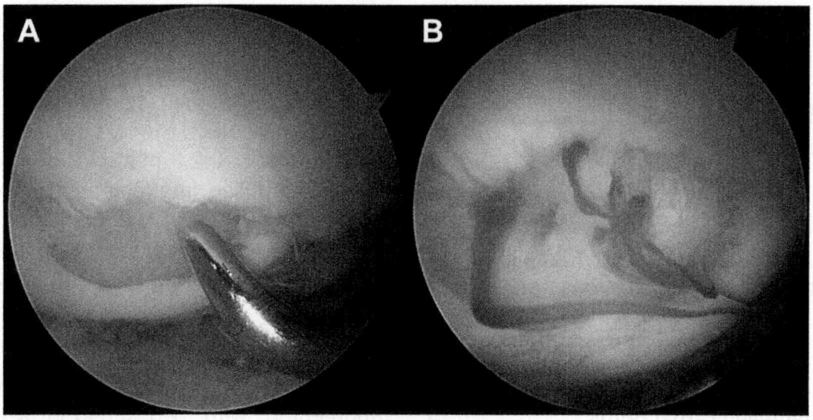

Fig. 5. Following chondroplasty to a stable edge, a microfracture awl is used to penetrate cortical bone (*A*), and the tourniquet is then released to confirm medullary bleeding (*B*).

lunate or triquetral microfracture in the literature, the authors' current practice for debridement of stable TFCC tears with microfracture of focal chondral lesions of the lunate and/or triquetrum has shown promising preliminary results.

Summary

Arthroscopic TFCC debridement and wafer resection seems to be a valuable treatment option for UIS and avoids the major pitfalls of USO, including high rates of hardware removal, risk of delayed union, and a more debilitating postoperative recovery period. Although larger prospective trials are needed, the best available evidence supports AWR and TFCC debridement as a viable treatment of UIS, especially in patients with less than 3 mm of ulnar positive variance. Microfracture is a promising technique to concomitantly treat chondral lesions within the lunate and triquetrum.

LUNOTRIQUETRAL INTEROSSEOUS LIGAMENT TEARS

LTIL tears may be seen in isolation or in association with other wrist pathology. Isolated LTIL injuries are thought to be caused by a fall on an outstretched hand in a pronated, extended, and radially deviated position.[61]

Clinical examination confirms tenderness over the lunotriquetral (LT) interval palpated just ulnar to the lunate in line with the fourth ray.[62] The LT ballottement test is performed by stabilizing the lunate and attempting to displace the triquetrum volarly and dorsally with a positive test reproducing pain, clicking, or laxity.[63–65] The Kleinman shuck test is performed with the lunate secured, and a dorsally directed load is placed on the pisotriquetral complex. As the wrist is brought into ulnar and radial deviation, a painful click is elicited in patients with an LTIL injury.[66] Plain radiographs should be obtained to look for carpal instability or a volar intercalated segmental instability (VISI) pattern. MRI with or without intraarticular contrast may further delineate pathoanatomy.

Indications/Contraindications

Arthroscopic treatment of LTIL tears is an option for injuries that have failed conservative management, such as casting and activity modification. Once operative treatment is decided on, the Geissler classification system, which grades LTIL tears based on instability with a probe in the LT joint, helps dictate appropriate treatment (**Table 1**).[67,68] The authors focus on arthroscopic treatment options, including debridement, thermal shrinkage capsulorraphy, and percutaneous pinning.

LTIL tears with a fixed VISI deformity are not amenable to arthroscopic stabilization procedures.

Surgical Approach

Step 1: The standard distraction tower and arthroscope are used. A complete radiocarpal and midcarpal diagnostic arthroscopy is performed, which should include the use of the 6R and ulnar midcarpal portals as viewing portals to completely visualize the LTIL from dorsal to palmar to check for its integrity and also the congruency of the lunate and triquetrum. Laxity should also be assessed on triquetral rotation and separation from the lunate.

Step 2: The treatment protocol for LTIL is based on the Geissler stage.

Table 1
Geissler grading for intercarpal ligament tears

Grade	Description
I	Attenuation or hemorrhage of interosseous ligament as seen from radiocarpal space; no incongruence of carpal alignment in midcarpal space
II	Attenuation or hemorrhage of interosseous ligament as seen from radiocarpal space; incongruence or step-off of carpal space; may be slight gap (less than width of probe) between carpal bones
III	Incongruence or step-off of carpal alignment as seen from both radiocarpal and midcarpal space; probe may be passed through gap between carpal bones
IV	Incongruence or step-off of carpal alignment as seen from both radiocarpal and midcarpal space; probe may be passed through gap between carpal bones

Data from Geissler WB, et al. Intracarpal soft-tissue lesions associated with an intra-articular fracture of the distal end of the radius. J Bone Joint Surg Am 1996;78(3):357–65.

Geissler stage I and II

For these injuries, simple debridement with or without thermal shrinkage is performed. Debridement of the torn edges of the ligament and synovitic tissue is performed with a 3.5-mm motorized shaver. Redundancy and tension of the remaining ligament is assessed.

Thermal shrinkage may be performed to tighten the remaining ligament. This procedure is performed using a modified technique described by Darlis and colleagues[69] in the setting of scapholunate ligament tears and by Lee and colleagues for LTIL tears.[70] A 2.3-mm bipolar radiofrequency probe is applied intermittently to the intact ligament in a paintbrush fashion from distal to proximal while visually confirming changes in color and consistency of the ligament (**Fig. 6**A, B).

Geissler stage III

These injuries may be treated with debridement and thermal shrinkage, however this should be augmented with two 0.045-in k-wires placed percutaneously using a modified technique described by Moskal and colleagues.[71] Reduction of the lunotriquetral joint is maintained while k-wires are placed under fluoroscopic guidance. In Geissler stage IV injuries, arthroscopic treatment is limited to the modalities described earlier. In this setting, more invasive procedures need to be considered, such as direct repair, reconstruction, arthrodesis, or ulnar shortening osteotomy.

Postoperative Care

The length of postoperative immobilization depends on the procedure that is performed. Following simple debridement, immobilization is discontinued after 2 weeks and therapy is begun. Following thermal shrinkage of the LTIL with or without pinning, patients are immobilized for 8 weeks in a short arm cast after which the pins are removed and therapy is begun. Strengthening begins at 12 weeks postoperatively, and full activity is typically restored at 4 months.

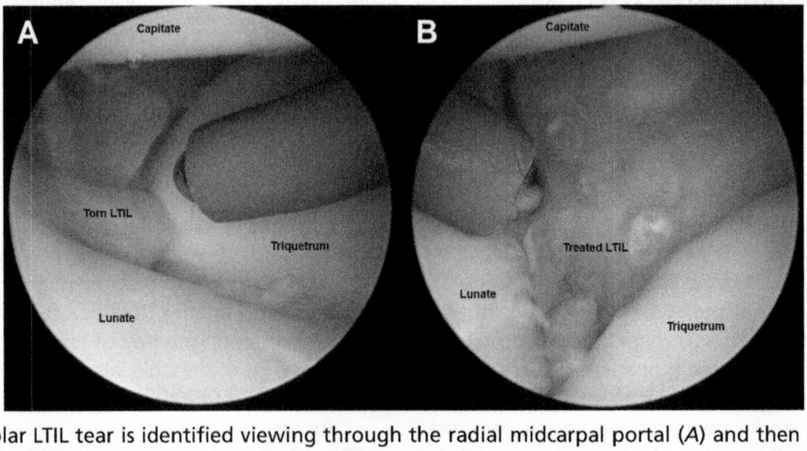

Fig. 6. The volar LTIL tear is identified viewing through the radial midcarpal portal (*A*) and then intermittently pulsed with the radiofrequency probe to achieve thermal shrinkage as seen via the ulnar midcarpal portal (*B*). The LT interval may be pinned with k-wires for 8 weeks to protect the stabilization.

Outcomes

Multiple studies have shown debridement alone may lead to symptomatic improvement in patients with both partial and complete LTIL tears. Weiss and colleagues[72] reported results on 6 patients with partial LTIL tears; all had complete or near complete resolution of pain at 27 months. Seven of 9 patients in their series with complete LTIL tears had complete resolution of their symptoms or only occasional symptoms following debridement alone.[72] Ruch and Poehling[73] reported that 13 of 14 patients were highly satisfied after debridement alone of SLIL or LTIL tears.[73] Westkaemper and colleagues,[40] however, reported poor results in 4 of 5 patients treated with debridement alone and attributed these outcomes to a lack of pinning the lunate and triquetrum.[40]

Osterman and Seidman[74] reported that LT debridement and pinning provided 80% of their patients with complete pain relief.[74] Moskal and colleagues[71] performed arthroscopic debridement, capsulodesis, and pinning of LTIL injuries and reported 18 of 20 patients with excellent or good results.[71] Lee and colleagues[70] described a technique of arthroscopic debridement and thermal shrinkage for SLIL and LTIL tears and reported a decrease in pain and good or excellent functional outcomes in 16 of 16 patients at greater than 4 years. Those researchers attributed their results to a combination of debridement, tightening of the LT ligament, and thermal denervation by the radiofrequency probe.[70]

Summary

Ulnar-sided wrist pain caused by LT interval pathology should typically undergo an initial period of nonoperative treatment. Options for arthroscopic treatment include debridement with or without thermal shrinkage and k-wire stabilization of the LT interval. These measures have been found to produce good short-term and midterm results. In the case of failure of these techniques, LTIL reconstruction, LT arthrodesis, or USO may be considered.

HAMATE ARTHROSIS

Proximal pole hamate arthrosis is a cause of ulnar-sided wrist pain seen commonly in patients who participate in sports with repetitive ulnar-deviation loading forces, such as golf. Although the cause of hamate arthrosis is likely multifactorial, anatomic variations in the lunate have been strongly correlated. Type I lunates have no articulation with the hamate and are found in 35% to 53% of wrists. Type II lunates have a medial articulation with the hamate and are found in 47% to 65% of wrists.[75,76] In anatomic studies, proximal pole hamate arthrosis was found almost exclusively in type II lunates, and motion analysis studies have demonstrated that contact between the hamate and lunate occurs only in type II lunates in ulnar deviation of the wrist.[76,77] Clinical studies have found a strong correlation between LTIL tears and hamate arthrosis, leading to the proposed acronym HALT (hamate arthrosis LTIL tear).[75,78] The abnormal kinematics seen with an LT dissociation may lead to abnormal loading at the triquetral-hamate joint, much like the development of radiocarpal arthrosis in the face of a chronic scapholunate ligament injury (scapholunate advanced collapse wrist). This abnormal loading may lead to arthrosis of the proximal pole of the hamate.

Although there is no physical examination finding that is pathognomonic for painful hamate arthrosis, patients should have pain with forced ulnar deviation and axial loading of the wrist. This maneuver will likely be positive in patients with pathology of the TFCC and/or ulnocarpal impaction; thus, the key in treatment is to recognize hamate arthrosis on preoperative imaging, correlate this with findings during arthroscopy, and treat as indicated by the pathology. Preoperative radiographs should demonstrate a type II lunate, with MRI more sensitive for the evaluation of chondral defects and subchondral bony edema (**Fig. 7**A).

Indications for Surgery

Proximal pole hamate arthritis refractory to conservative management is an excellent indication for arthroscopic debridement in the form of chondroplasty or proximal pole excision. Arthroscopy is particularly advantageous because it allows the surgeon to address any concomitant pathology.

Surgical Technique

The standard distraction tower and arthroscope are used. Diagnostic midcarpal arthroscopy is performed confirming proximal hamate arthrosis while paying attention to the LT interval and TFCC (see **Fig. 7**B). With the arthroscope in the radial midcarpal portal, a 2.9-mm burr is inserted into the ulnar midcarpal portal (see **Fig. 7**C). An average of 2.4 mm of the proximal pole should be excised because that has been shown to be adequate to fully unload the hamatolunate articulation while leaving loads across the triquetrohamate joint unaltered (see **Fig. 7**D). To fully excise the proximal pole of the hamate, the portals may need to be switched. Microfracture for chondral

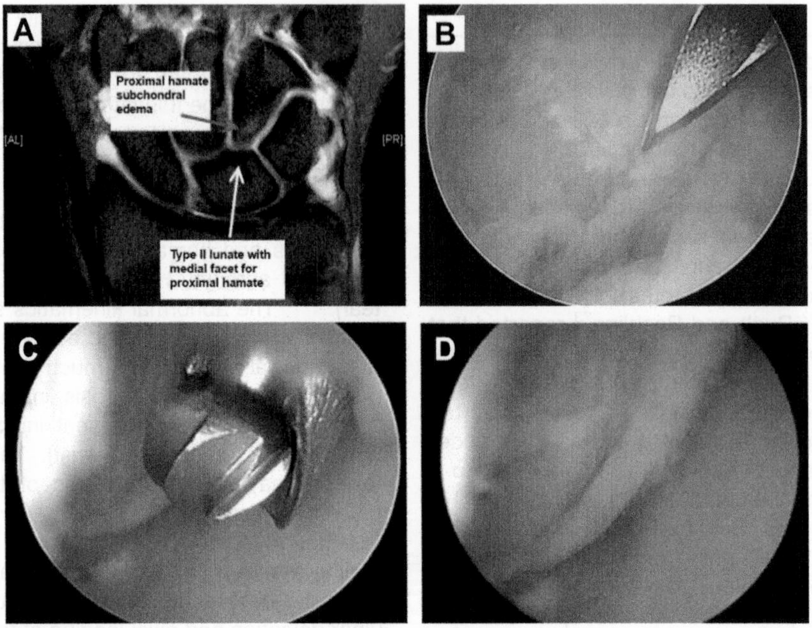

Fig. 7. Representative MRI demonstrating a type II lunate with proximal hamate arthrosis (*A*) with arthroscopic confirmation (*B*) followed by use of 2.9-mm burr (*C*) to resect approximately 2.4 mm of proximal hamate (*D*).

defects of the proximal pole of the hamate may also be a viable treatment alternative.

Postoperative Care

Postoperatively, patients are placed in a volar-based short arm splint for 7 to 10 days, after which they return for a wound check and suture removal. Immediate wrist motion is encouraged, with protection against vigorous activity for 6 weeks.

Outcomes

Harley and colleagues[78] reported 86% good to excellent results with arthroscopic proximal pole of hamate excision, removing an average of 2.2 mm. Seventy-eight percent of the patients in that study had a rapid return to work, and results did not deteriorate significantly over an average of 4.7 years of follow-up. The patients with poor outcomes had multiple concomitant injuries. It is a benefit of arthroscopy, however, that these diagnoses may be made at the time of the index procedure, and the patients' prognosis may be predicted.

Summary

Patients with a type II lunate who perform activities with ulnar-deviation loading forces may be predisposed to develop proximal pole hamate arthritis. The extent to which lunotriquetral instability contributes in the development of hamate arthrosis is not fully understood, but a strong correlation has been shown. Arthroscopic proximal pole hamate excision of at least 2.2 to 2.4 mm is an excellent treatment option for these patients with this cause of ulnar-sided wrist pain.

SUMMARY

Ulnar-sided wrist pain is a common cause of pain and disability, which has long been a diagnostic and therapeutic dilemma for hand surgeons. A thorough understanding of the anatomy, clinical examination, and radiographic evaluation is essential to establish a focused differential diagnosis, with the cause of disability often being multifactorial. Arthroscopy is particularly well suited to both directly visualize and treat multiple causes of ulnar-sided wrist pain, including pathology of the TFCC, UIS, LTIL tears, and hamate arthrosis.

REFERENCES

1. Palmer AK. Triangular fibrocartilage disorders: injury patterns and treatment. Arthroscopy 1990; 6(2):125–32.
2. Palmer AK, Glisson RR, Werner FW. Relationship between ulnar variance and triangular fibrocartilage complex thickness. J Hand Surg Am 1984; 9(5):681–2.
3. Palmer AK, Werner FW. The triangular fibrocartilage complex of the wrist–anatomy and function. J Hand Surg Am 1981;6(2):153–62.

4. Palmer AK, Werner FW. Biomechanics of the distal radioulnar joint. Clin Orthop Relat Res 1984;(187): 26–35.
5. Palmer AK, Werner FW, Glisson RR, et al. Partial excision of the triangular fibrocartilage complex. J Hand Surg Am 1988;13(3):391–4.
6. McAdams TR, Swan J, Yao J. Arthroscopic treatment of triangular fibrocartilage wrist injuries in the athlete. Am J Sports Med 2009;37(2):291–7.
7. Tay SC, Tomita K, Berger RA. The "ulnar fovea sign" for defining ulnar wrist pain: an analysis of sensitivity and specificity. J Hand Surg Am 2007; 32(4):438–44.
8. Nakamura R, Horii E, Imaeda T, et al. The ulnocarpal stress test in the diagnosis of ulnar-sided wrist pain. J Hand Surg Br 1997;22(6):719–23.
9. Blazar PE, Chan PS, Kneeland JB, et al. The effect of observer experience on magnetic resonance imaging interpretation and localization of triangular fibrocartilage complex lesions. J Hand Surg Am 2001;26(4):742–8.
10. Potter HG, Asnis-Ernberg L, Weiland AJ, et al. The utility of high-resolution magnetic resonance imaging in the evaluation of the triangular fibrocartilage complex of the wrist. J Bone Joint Surg Am 1997; 79(11):1675–84.
11. Friedman SL, Palmer AK. The ulnar impaction syndrome. Hand Clin 1991;7(2):295–310.
12. Palmer AK. Triangular fibrocartilage complex lesions: a classification. J Hand Surg Am 1989; 14(4):594–606.
13. Adams BD. Partial excision of the triangular fibrocartilage complex articular disk: a biomechanical study. J Hand Surg Am 1993;18(2):334–40.
14. Park MJ, Jagadish A, Yao J. The rate of triangular fibrocartilage injuries requiring surgical intervention. Orthopedics 2010;33(11):806.
15. Minami A, Ishikawa J, Suenaga N, et al. Clinical results of treatment of triangular fibrocartilage complex tears by arthroscopic debridement. J Hand Surg Am 1996;21(3):406–11.
16. Bernstein MA, Nagle DJ, Martinez A, et al. A comparison of combined arthroscopic triangular fibrocartilage complex debridement and arthroscopic wafer distal ulna resection versus arthroscopic triangular fibrocartilage complex debridement and ulnar shortening osteotomy for ulnocarpal abutment syndrome. Arthroscopy 2004;20(4):392–401.
17. Hulsizer D, Weiss AP, Akelman E. Ulna-shortening osteotomy after failed arthroscopic debridement of the triangular fibrocartilage complex. J Hand Surg Am 1997;22(4):694–8.
18. Ruch DS, Papadonikolakis A. Arthroscopically assisted repair of peripheral triangular fibrocartilage complex tears: factors affecting outcome. Arthroscopy 2005;21(9):1126–30.
19. Bednar MS, Arnoczky SP, Weiland AJ. The microvasculature of the triangular fibrocartilage complex: its clinical significance. J Hand Surg Am 1991;16(6):1101–5.
20. Yao J, Dantuluri P, Osterman AL. A novel technique of all-inside arthroscopic triangular fibrocartilage complex repair. Arthroscopy 2007;23(12):1357. e1–4.
21. Yao J, Lee AT. All-arthroscopic repair of Palmer 1B triangular fibrocartilage complex tears using the FasT-Fix device. J Hand Surg Am 2011;36(5): 836–42.
22. Yao J. All-arthroscopic repair of peripheral triangular fibrocartilage complex tears using FasT-Fix. Hand Clin 2011;27(3):237–42.
23. de Araujo W, Poehling GG, Kuzma GR. New Tuohy needle technique for triangular fibrocartilage complex repair: preliminary studies. Arthroscopy 1996; 12(6):699–703.
24. Estrella EP, Hung LK, Ho PC, et al. Arthroscopic repair of triangular fibrocartilage complex tears. Arthroscopy 2007;23(7):729–37, 737.e1.
25. Geissler WB. Arthroscopic knotless peripheral triangular fibrocartilage repair. J Hand Surg Am 2012;37(2):350–5.
26. Pederzini LA, Tosi M, Prandini M, et al. All-inside suture technique for Palmer class 1B triangular fibrocartilage repair. Arthroscopy 2007;23(10): 1130.e1–4.
27. Trumble TE, Gilbert M, Vedder N. Arthroscopic repair of the triangular fibrocartilage complex. Arthroscopy 1996;12(5):588–97.
28. Tay SC, Berger RA, Parker WL. Longitudinal split tears of the ulnotriquetral ligament. Hand Clin 2010;26(4):495–501.
29. Thiru RG, Ferlic DC, Clayton ML, et al. Arterial anatomy of the triangular fibrocartilage of the wrist and its surgical significance. J Hand Surg Am 1986; 11(2):258–63.
30. Sagerman SD, Short W. Arthroscopic repair of radial-sided triangular fibrocartilage complex tears. Arthroscopy 1996;12(3):339–42.
31. Wolf MB, Kroeber MW, Reiter A, et al. Ulnar shortening after TFCC suture repair of Palmer type 1B lesions. Arch Orthop Trauma Surg 2010;130(3): 301–6.
32. Atzei A, Luchetti R. Foveal TFCC tear classification and treatment. Hand Clin 2011;27(3):263–72.
33. Iwasaki N, Nishida K, Motomiya M, et al. Arthroscopic-assisted repair of avulsed triangular fibrocartilage complex to the fovea of the ulnar head: a 2- to 4-year follow-up study. Arthroscopy 2011; 27(10):1371–8.
34. Tang CY, Fung B, Rebecca C, et al. Another light in the dark: review of a new method for the arthroscopic repair of triangular fibrocartilage complex. J Hand Surg Am 2012;37(6):1263–8.

35. Yao J. All-arthroscopic triangular fibrocartilage complex repair: safety and biomechanical comparison with a traditional outside-in technique in cadavers. J Hand Surg Am 2009;34(4):671–6.
36. Darlis NA, Weiser RW, Sotereanos DG. Arthroscopic triangular fibrocartilage complex debridement using radiofrequency probes. J Hand Surg Br 2005;30(6):638–42.
37. Husby T, Haugstvedt JR. Long-term results after arthroscopic resection of lesions of the triangular fibrocartilage complex. Scand J Plast Reconstr Surg Hand Surg 2001;35(1):79–83.
38. Infanger M, Grimm D. Meniscus and discus lesions of triangular fibrocartilage complex (TFCC): treatment by laser-assisted wrist arthroscopy. J Plast Reconstr Aesthet Surg 2009;62(4):466–71.
39. Miwa H, Hashizume H, Fujiwara K, et al. Arthroscopic surgery for traumatic triangular fibrocartilage complex injury. J Orthop Sci 2004;9(4):354–9.
40. Westkaemper JG, Mitsionis G, Giannakopoulos PN, et al. Wrist arthroscopy for the treatment of ligament and triangular fibrocartilage complex injuries. Arthroscopy 1998;14(5):479–83.
41. Anderson ML, Larson AN, Moran SL, et al. Clinical comparison of arthroscopic versus open repair of triangular fibrocartilage complex tears. J Hand Surg Am 2008;33(5):675–82.
42. Millants P, De Smet L, Van Ransbeeck H. Outcome study of arthroscopic suturing of ulnar avulsions of the triangular fibrocartilage complex of the wrist. Chir Main 2002;21(5):298–300.
43. Corso SJ, Savoie FH, Geissler WB, et al. Arthroscopic repair of peripheral avulsions of the triangular fibrocartilage complex of the wrist: a multicenter study. Arthroscopy 1997;13(1):78–84.
44. Wolf MB, Haas A, Dragu A, et al. Arthroscopic repair of ulnar-sided triangular fibrocartilage complex (Palmer type 1B) tears: a comparison between short- and midterm results. J Hand Surg Am 2012;37(11):2325–30.
45. Nakamura T, Sato K, Okazaki M, et al. Repair of foveal detachment of the triangular fibrocartilage complex: open and arthroscopic transosseous techniques. Hand Clin 2011;27(3):281–90.
46. Shinohara T, Tatebe M, Okui N, et al. Arthroscopically assisted repair of triangular fibrocartilage complex foveal tears. J Hand Surg Am 2013;38(2):271–7.
47. Cardenas-Montemayor E, Hartl JF, Wolf MB, et al. Subjective and objective results of arthroscopic debridement of ulnar-sided TFCC (Palmer type 1B) lesions with stable distal radio-ulnar joint. Arch Orthop Trauma Surg 2013;133(2):287–93.
48. Trumble TE, Gilbert M, Vedder N. Isolated tears of the triangular fibrocartilage: management by early arthroscopic repair. J Hand Surg Am 1997;22(1):57–65.
49. Bickel KD. Arthroscopic treatment of ulnar impaction syndrome. J Hand Surg Am 2008;33(8):1420–3.
50. Constantine KJ, Tomaino MM, Herndon JH, et al. Comparison of ulnar shortening osteotomy and the wafer resection procedure as treatment for ulnar impaction syndrome. J Hand Surg Am 2000;25(1):55–60.
51. Feldon P, Terrono AL, Belsky MR. Wafer distal ulna resection for triangular fibrocartilage tears and/or ulna impaction syndrome. J Hand Surg Am 1992;17(4):731–7.
52. Loftus JB. Arthroscopic wafer for ulnar impaction syndrome. Tech Hand Up Extrem Surg 2000;4(3):182–8.
53. Nagle DJ, Bernstein MA. Laser-assisted arthroscopic ulnar shortening. Arthroscopy 2002;18(9):1046–51.
54. Adams BD, Holley KA. Strains in the articular disk of the triangular fibrocartilage complex: a biomechanical study. J Hand Surg Am 1993;18(5):919–25.
55. Stuart PR, Berger RA, Linscheid RL, et al. The dorsopalmar stability of the distal radioulnar joint. J Hand Surg Am 2000;25(4):689–99.
56. Tomaino MM, Weiser RW. Combined arthroscopic TFCC debridement and wafer resection of the distal ulna in wrists with triangular fibrocartilage complex tears and positive ulnar variance. J Hand Surg Am 2001;26(6):1047–52.
57. De Smet L, De Ferm A, Steenwerckx A, et al. Arthroscopic treatment of triangular fibrocartilage complex lesions of the wrist. Acta Orthop Belg 1996;62(1):8–13.
58. Meftah M, Keefer EP, Panagopoulos, et al. Arthroscopic wafer resection for ulnar impaction syndrome: prediction of outcomes. Hand Surg 2010;15(2):89–93.
59. Osterman AL. Arthroscopic debridement of triangular fibrocartilage complex tears. Arthroscopy 1990;6(2):120–4.
60. Vandenberghe L, Degreef I, Didden K, et al. Ulnar shortening or arthroscopic wafer resection for ulnar impaction syndrome. Acta Orthop Belg 2012;78(3):323–6.
61. Shin AY, Weinstein LP, Berger RA, et al. Treatment of isolated injuries of the lunotriquetral ligament. A comparison of arthrodesis, ligament reconstruction and ligament repair. J Bone Joint Surg Br 2001;83(7):1023–8.
62. Ambrose L, Posner MA. Lunate-triquetral and midcarpal joint instability. Hand Clin 1992;8(4):653–68.
63. Mayfield JK. Patterns of injury to carpal ligaments. A spectrum. Clin Orthop Relat Res 1984;(187):36–42.
64. Reagan DS, Linscheid RL, Dobyns JH. Lunotriquetral sprains. J Hand Surg Am 1984;9(4):502–14.

65. Skirven T. Clinical examination of the wrist. J Hand Ther 1996;9(2):96–107.
66. Bednar JM, Osterman AL. Carpal instability: evaluation and treatment. J Am Acad Orthop Surg 1993; 1(1):10–7.
67. Chloros GD, Wiesler ER, Poehling GG. Current concepts in wrist arthroscopy. Arthroscopy 2008; 24(3):343–54.
68. Geissler WB, Freeland AE, Savoie FH, et al. Intracarpal soft-tissue lesions associated with an intraarticular fracture of the distal end of the radius. J Bone Joint Surg Am 1996;78(3):357–65.
69. Darlis NA, Weiser RW, Sotereanos DG. Partial scapholunate ligament injuries treated with arthroscopic debridement and thermal shrinkage. J Hand Surg Am 2005;30(5):908–14.
70. Lee JI, Nha KW, Lee GY, et al. Long-term outcomes of arthroscopic debridement and thermal shrinkage for isolated partial intercarpal ligament tears. Orthopedics 2012;35(8):e1204–9.
71. Moskal MJ, Savoie FH 3rd, Field LD. Arthroscopic capsulodesis of the lunotriquetral joint. Clin Sports Med 2001;20(1):141–53, ix–x.
72. Weiss AP, Sachar K, Glowacki KA. Arthroscopic debridement alone for intercarpal ligament tears. J Hand Surg Am 1997;22(2):344–9.
73. Ruch DS, Poehling GG. Arthroscopic management of partial scapholunate and lunotriquetral injuries of the wrist. J Hand Surg Am 1996;21(3): 412–7.
74. Osterman AL, Seidman GD. The role of arthroscopy in the treatment of lunatotriquetral ligament injuries. Hand Clin 1995;11(1):41–50.
75. Burgess RC. Anatomic variations of the midcarpal joint. J Hand Surg Am 1990;15(1):129–31.
76. Viegas SF, Wagner SF, Patterson R, et al. Medial (hamate) facet of the lunate. J Hand Surg Am 1990;15(4):564–71.
77. Nakamura K, Beppu M, Patterson RM, et al. Motion analysis in two dimensions of radial-ulnar deviation of type I versus type II lunates. J Hand Surg Am 2000;25(5):877–88.
78. Harley BJ, Werner FW, Boles SD, et al. Arthroscopic resection of arthrosis of the proximal hamate: a clinical and biomechanical study. J Hand Surg Am 2004;29(4):661–7.

Use of Arthroscopy for the Treatment of Scaphoid Fractures

David J. Slutsky, MD[a,*], Julien Trevare[b]

KEYWORDS

• Scaphoid • Arthroscopy • Fracture • Nonunion

KEY POINTS

- An arthroscopic assist for scaphoid fixation is useful to assess the quality of the reduction, the stability of fixation, and to assess hardware position.
- Arthroscopy allows one to evaluate and treat any associated ligament injuries.
- Scaphoid waist fractures can be treated with either a volar or dorsal approach. Distal scaphoid fractures are managed with a retrograde screw insertion, whereas proximal pole fractures are treated with an antegrade screw insertion.
- Specialized training in wrist arthroscopy is desirable before attempting an arthroscopic assisted screw fixation.

INTRODUCTION: NATURE OF THE PROBLEM

Minimally invasive approaches are increasingly popular in the treatment of hand fractures. For scaphoid fractures, decreasing the incision size and limiting the dissection have lead to the adoption of percutaneous approaches. Most scaphoid screws are well positioned using a percutaneous or mini-open approach. However, these small incisions can limit the surgeon's ability to fully understand the anatomy and assess the reduction. In these instances, arthroscopic assist can be advantageous ensuring better implant placement and a more predictable result. Specifically, arthroscopy can aid optimal guidewire positioning. Arthroscopy allows direct visualization of the fracture even with minimal skin incisions, which allows assessment of the quality of fracture reduction, especially for comminuted fractures. Arthroscopy provides evaluation of the rigidity of fixation, because seemingly good screw purchase may not adequately stabilize a comminuted segment. One can use arthroscopic techniques to assess screw length and ensure there is no radiocarpal penetration with retrograde (volar) insertion or conversely to check that the screw threads are well buried in the proximal pole with dorsal (antegrade) insertion. Finally, scaphoid fractures can have associated ligamentous injuries, and arthroscopy allows the surgeon to evaluate for other potential soft tissue injuries.[1]

INDICATIONS/CONTRAINDICATIONS

Indications

The indications for percutaneous screw fixation parallel those for an open reduction. These indications include any acute proximal pole fracture or any reducible scaphoid waist fracture with more than 1 mm of displacement or translation. Angulated fractures and fractures with significant comminution as well as combined injuries can also be managed with percutaneous reduction and fixation, but these are the type of cases that would benefit from an arthroscopic assist. Nondisplaced fibrous scaphoid nonunions without evidence of avascular necrosis are also suitable candidates for percutaneous fixation. Acute

[a] Department of Orthopedics, Harbor-UCLA Medical Center, The Hand and Wrist Institute, 2808 Columbia Street, Torrance, CA 90503, USA; [b] Culver City, CA, USA
* Corresponding author.
E-mail address: d-slutsky@msn.com

Hand Clin 30 (2014) 91–103
http://dx.doi.org/10.1016/j.hcl.2013.09.002

nondisplaced scaphoid waist fractures can be effectively treated with cast immobilization; however, there are some instances where screw fixation is considered such as high performance athlete, economic hardship with prolonged casting, or patients who cannot tolerate immobilization for psychological reasons. An arthroscopic assist allows the surgeon to use the percutaneous approach for more complex cases such as comminuted scaphoid fractures and when there is a suspicion of an associated ligament injury.

Contraindications

There are cases in which percutaneous approaches even with arthroscopic assist are not appropriate. Partial or complete avascular necrosis of the scaphoid is a relative contraindication, although Slade described healing of avascular proximal using percutaneous methods.[2] A very small proximal pole fragment does not allow adequate screw purchase and needs an alternative approach. Nonunions with a humpback deformity and a secondary dorsal intercalated segmental instability (DISI) pattern usually require an open volar wedge graft, which requires wide exposure. An alternative approach is required in the presence of significant radiocarpal and/or midcarpal degenerative changes. Finally, arthroscopy is contraindicated in the presence of active infection, bleeding disorders, or a poor skin envelope.

SURGICAL TECHNIQUE

Preoperative Planning

Approach

After the decision for surgical intervention, the next step is to decide what is the best approach as the implant can be placed through either dorsally or volarly. The dorsal technique has the disadvantage of creating a hole in the weight-bearing surface of the proximal scaphoid pole but it allows more direct access to the central axis of the scaphoid. Dorsal screw insertion is the recommended approach for proximal pole fractures because this provides maximum fracture compression of the smaller proximal fragment. The volar approach is best for distal pole fractures. Volar implantation often requires eccentric screw placement through the distal pole, and there is limited area for screw insertion. To place the screw using the volar approach, the surgeon often has to ream through the trapezium to gain access to the central scaphoid axis. However, with careful planning, the volar approach allows the screw to be placed centrally through the waist and proximal pole.[3] An advantage of the volar technique is that the articular defect from the entry site is limited to the radial edge of the scaphotrapezial joint. Either dorsal or volar approach is used for a scaphoid waist fracture. A recent comparison of the volar and dorsal percutaneous screw fixation showed no difference in the ultimate union rates, although dorsal screw fixation tended to be closer to the central axis and more perpendicular to the fracture line with waist fractures.[4] In the end, the surgeon must evaluate the fracture and decide which approach best fits the patient and the fracture.

Imaging

Imaging is a necessary adjunct in both the preoperative planning and post-operative assessments of scaphoid fractures. Preoperatively the position of the fracture or the nonunion is assessed with anteroposterior (AP), lateral, and semipronated oblique wrist radiographs. A preoperative computed tomographic (CT) scan is helpful in difficult cases and has become the gold standard in assessing the degree of bony union post-operatively. With a longstanding nonunion, the author practices to perform a preoperative magnetic resonance imaging (MRI) in all cases to rule out avascular necrosis of the proximal fragment.

Screw placement

An essential component to success in the operative scaphoid fracture treatment is proper placement of the screw. The implant should be placed down the central axis of the scaphoid as this position provides the greatest rigidity.[5] Correct positioning results in faster union rates and allows longer screw insertion, which better distributes the bending forces.[6] Because guidewire insertion and screw placement are the critical steps of the procedure, several researchers have attempted to quantify the optimum starting position for screw insertion so that the screw ends up in the central one-third of the proximal pole.[7] Menapace and colleagues[8] defined a safe zone for volar k-wire insertion for placement of a Herbert-Whipple screw based on radiograph, CT, and anatomic dissections. To limit the risk of damaging the scaphoid blood supply, they recommended avoidance of the radiodorsal portion of the scaphoid (provides 70%–80% of the blood supply) and the volar surface of the scaphoid tuberosity (provides 20%–30% of the blood supply). They also eschewed the ulnar one-third of the scaphoid so that the scaphocapitate articulation was not compromised. They also noted that paired scaphoids had no significant radiographic differences in the lengths and widths, allowing the contralateral scaphoid to be a measuring template for screw placement planning. After reviewing their results, they defined the safe starting point to be 4 to 5 mm dorsal and distal to the volar prominence of the tubercle. The ideal targeting point for the screw point was 10% of the radiographic length of the contralateral scaphoid, which equated to 2 to 3 mm in a radial and slightly volar direction from the central part of the scapholunate interosseous ligament.

Leventhal and colleagues[9] performed a CT study of 9 scaphoids. They computed a safe zone that was located 2.3 mm inside the original cortical bone surface, based on a 1.7 mm screw radius (Acutrak 2 Mini; Acumed LLC, Hillsboro, OR), an 0.035 mm cortical bone thickness, and an additional 0.25 mm safety margin. They found that the central axis was partially or completely obstructed by the trapezium in all specimens. When they looked at the longitudinal axis that allowed them to place the maximum length screw, they found the safe zone passed on average 1.8 mm ± 0.8 mm away in primarily a dorsal and slightly radial direction (0.2 mm) from the apex of the scaphoid tubercle and exited ulnar and slightly dorsal to the longitudinal axis. They did acknowledge that placing the wrist in traction and ulnar deviation might provide greater access by further increasing the distance from the screw axis to the trapezium. Use of a larger diameter screw would also change these findings.

Arthroscopic portals

There are several portals that are useful when treating scaphoid fractures.

The scaphotrapezial trapezoidal (STT)-U portal is located in line with the midshaft axis of the index metacarpal, just ulnar to the extensor pollicus longus tendon.

The STT-R portal is radial to the abductor pollicus longus tendon at the level of the STT joint.

The MCU is the midcarpal ulnar portal, which is located 1 cm distal to the 4,5 portal in line with the ring finger.

The MCR is the midcarpal radial portal, which is located 1 cm distal to the 3,4 portal in line with the index finger.

SURGICAL PROCEDURE

Dorsal Approach

Step 1

The patient is positioned supine on the operating room table with the arm abducted on a hand table. The fluoroscopy unit is positioned over the arm board, parallel to the floor. The ARC traction tower (ARC Medical, Beaverton, OR) is ideally suited for this procedure because it has no central pole to obstruct instrumentation, and the wrist can be flexed to 45° in traction, which allows one to alternate between a fluoroscopic and arthroscopic assessment without moving the C-arm or extending the wrist (**Fig. 1**). Alternatively the wrist is flexed 45° over folded towels, which places the scaphoid axis at 90° to the beam and facilitates placing the screw down the central axis.

Step 2

Guide wire insertion is accomplished percutaneously using fluoroscope control, initially without tourniquet. Antegrade screw insertion is used for proximal pole fractures because it provides the maximum bony purchase of small proximal pole fragments and it is easier to place the screw centrally than from a retrograde approach. The reverse is true for a distal pole fracture. Waist fractures can be treated with either approach while still placing the screw down the central axis.

Step 3

I hand insert 2 k-wires into the midline of the scaphotrapezial trapezoidal (STT) joint to act as targeting aids for guidewire insertion. The first guidewire is placed through the ulnar (STT-U) arthroscopy. The second guidewire is inserted through a radial portal (STT-R). The targeting wires should intersect at the midpoint of the STT joint. The ideal starting point for the guidewire is at the most proximal tip of the scaphoid pole immediately adjacent to the insertion of scapholunate interosseous ligament (SLIL). The third k-wire is placed into the dorsal aspect of the scapholunate interval just ulnar to this point. Alternatively, with the scope in the 3/4 or 4/5 portal, the tip of the

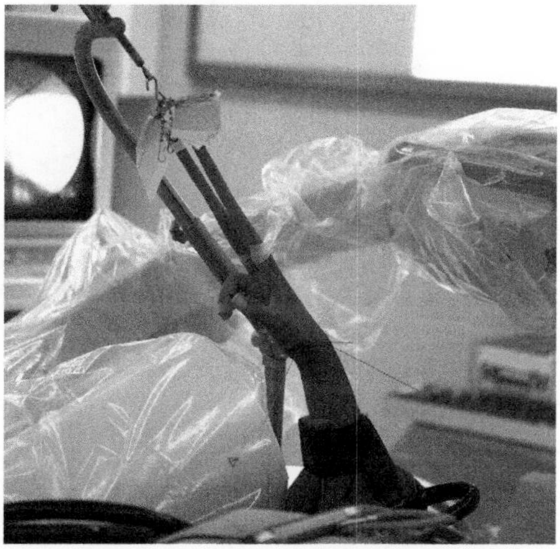

Fig. 1. Arthroscopic setup. The wrist is placed in traction and flexed 45° with a mini-fluoroscopy unit centered over the radiocarpal joint. This facilitates switching between arthroscopy and fluoroscopy without taking the wrist out of traction. (© 2013. Slutsky. All Rights Reserved.)

guidewire can be directed to the soft spot on the proximal pole bordering the SLIL insertion.

Step 4

Using a power drill, the guidewire is driven from an ulnar dorsal to a radial volar direction while keeping the wrist flexed. Aiming toward the intersection point of the dorsal STT k-wire on an AP fluoroscopic view guides the medial/lateral alignment of the guidewire. Pointing toward the intersection point of the radial STT k-wire on the semipronated fluoroscopic view guides the dorsal/volar alignment. The guidewire is then advanced distally through the trapezium and out through the skin (**Fig. 2**). The wrist can be extended if necessary once the trailing end clears the radiocarpal joint. If the fracture is displaced, the guidewire is withdrawn distally until it lies solely within the distal fragment.

Step 5

Percutaneous 0.62 mm k-wires can then be inserted into the proximal and distal fragments and used as joysticks to align the scaphoid. The

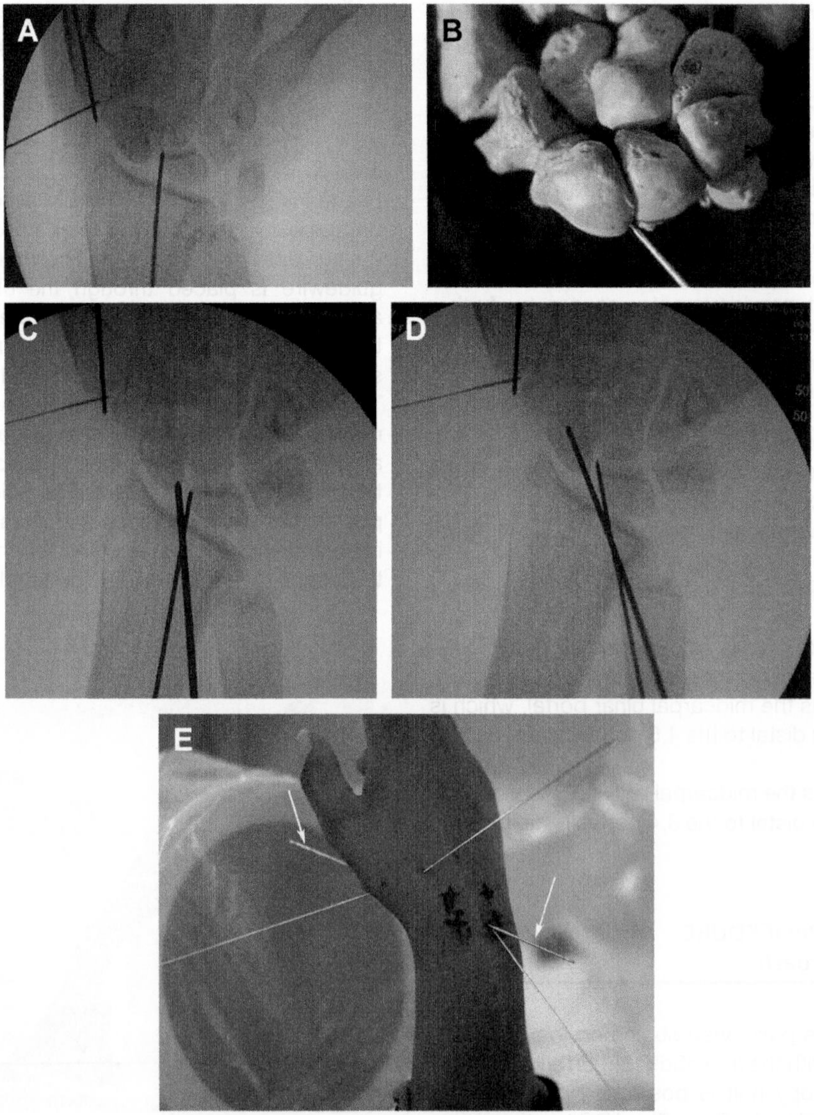

Fig. 2. K-wire targeting. (*A*) K-wires have been inserted in the scaphotrapezial joint in the coronal and sagittal planes. A third k-wire is placed in the scapholunate interval, which guides the starting point of the guidewire in the proximal pole. (*B*) A dry bone model demonstrating the ideal starting point for the guidewire in the proximal pole. (*C*) Guidewire is placed at the ulnar tip of the proximal pole. (*D*) Guidewire is advanced aiming toward the targeting k-wires. (*E*) Clinical photo. Note that the guidewire has been advanced through the trapezium and out of volar radial aspect of the thumb before reaming (*arrows*). (© 2013. Slutsky. All Rights Reserved.)

alignment of the concave scaphoid surface on the AP radiographic view can be used as a reference for fracture reduction. Once it is satisfactory, the reduction is captured by driving the guidewire proximally.

Step 6

The second antirotation k-wire should be inserted before reaming. The targeting k-wires are removed, and the reamer is then introduced over the guidewire. Reaming stops 2 mm short of the distal pole.

Step 7

The arm is exsanguinated and the tourniquet is elevated at this point. When using some other type of traction tower, the arm is suspended with 10 to 15 lbs of traction with the wrist in extension, and the quality of the fracture site reduction is visualized by inserting the arthroscope into the MCU portal with the probe in the MCR portal (**Fig. 3**). Adjustments to the fracture reduction can be performed by withdrawing the guidewire into the distal fragment and using a freer elevator alternately inserted in the MCR and STT-U portals.

Step 8

Once the reduction is acceptable, the guidewire is advanced to capture the reduction and positioned within 2 mm of the STT joint with the wrist maintained in flexion. Any associated intracarpal pathology should be addressed at this time and treated accordingly either with arthroscopic or open procedures.

Step 9

Most of the screw-measuring guides from different types of headless screws overestimate the screw length, hence a second wire of equal length is placed percutaneously on to the cortex of the proximal scaphoid pole and parallel to the guidewire. The difference in length between the trailing ends of each wire is the scaphoid length. The screw length selected should be 4 mm less than the scaphoid length, which permits 2 mm of clearance of the screw at each end of the scaphoid, thus ensuring complete implantation without screw exposure. If it is necessary to take the wrist out of traction for this part, the screw length can be gauged by driving the guidewire volarly and distally until the trailing end is in the subchondral bone of the distal scaphoid pole and the process is repeated. A recent anthropometric study by Bindra determined that the average scaphoid length in adult men was 31.3 $\pm$ 2.1 mm, whereas the average female scaphoid was 27.3 $\pm$ 1.7 mm, hence the longest screw lengths may range from 23 mm to 27 mm.[10]

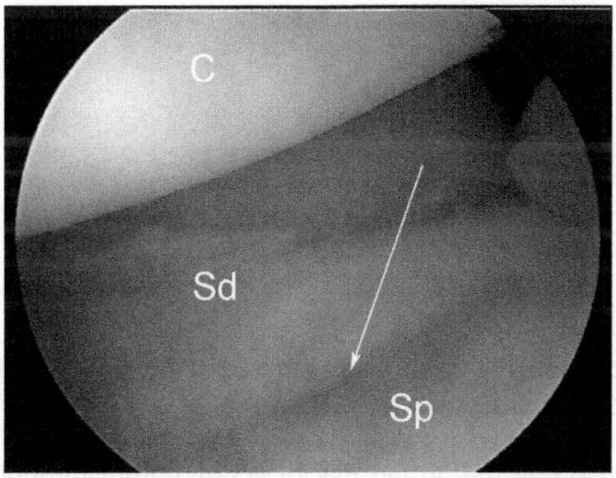

Fig. 3. View of a reduced scaphoid fracture (*arrow*) from the midcarpal ulnar portal. C, capitate; Sd, scaphoid distal pole; Sp, scaphoid proximal pole. (© 2013. Slutsky. All Rights Reserved.)

Step 10

After the length of the screw has been calculated, the guidewire is driven volarly once more so that it is left protruding both proximally and distally; this prevents guidewire migration during reaming and screw insertion. The wrist must remain flexed during this part otherwise the guidewire will bend and block both reaming and screw insertion.

Step 11

The scaphoid is then power reamed to within 2 mm of the distal pole. Care is taken not to ream through the subchondral bone because this reduces compression along the fracture site. A headless screw is advanced under fluoroscopic guidance to within 1 to 2 mm of the opposite cortex.

Step 12

Radiocarpal and midcarpal arthroscopy is now performed to check for screw cut out. The rigidity of fracture fixation is assessed by palpating the fragments with a 1-mm hook probe or freer elevator. After screw insertion, the guidewire is again driven distally if necessary to allow wrist extension, and the fracture site is inspected arthroscopically. If rigid fixation has not been achieved, Slade has recommended pinning the distal fragment to the capitate (**Fig. 4**)[11]; this locks the midcarpal row and reduces fracture site motion, especially with short proximal or distal fragments where only a few screw threads cross the fracture site. If desired, percutaneous iliac bone graft harvested with a bone biopsy needle or demineralized bone matrix can be injected percutaneously by advancing the arthroscopic cannula down the guidewire and into the drill hole in the proximal scaphoid, before screw insertion.

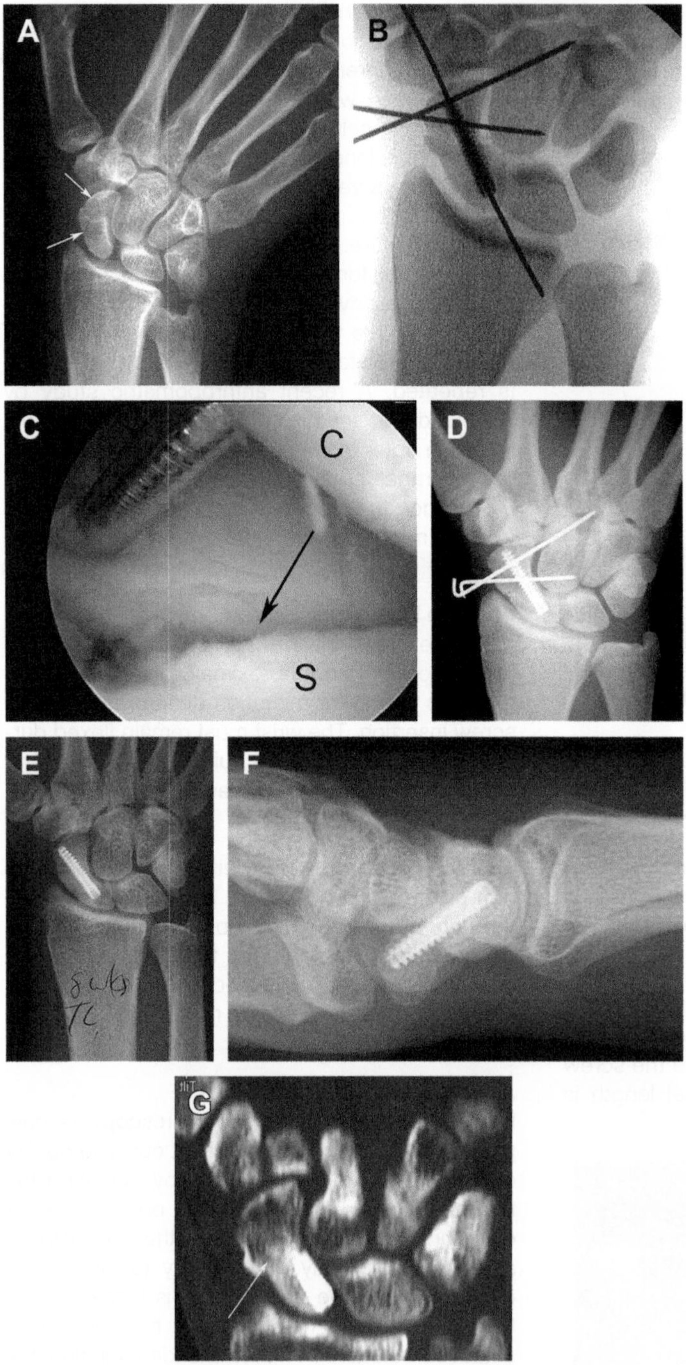

Fig. 4. (*A*) Comminuted scaphoid fracture with 2 fracture lines (*arrows*). (*B*) The comminuted segment is k-wired to the capitate to block fracture site motion. (*C*) Arthroscopic view from the midcarpal radial portal of the k-wire and comminuted segment (*arrow*). (*D*) Completed construct. (*E, F*) Radiographic signs of fracture union at 8 weeks. Ideal screw length is 2 mm from both poles. (*G*) CT scan demonstrating bridging callus at the fracture site (*arrow*). (© 2013. Slutsky. All Rights Reserved.)

Volar Approach

Preoperative planning

As a general rule, volar implantation is ideal for distal pole and scaphoid waist fractures. Volar implantation requires eccentric screw placement because of the need to ream through the trapezium to gain access to the scaphoid. Despite this oblique distal starting point, the screw can still be placed down the central canal at the level of the waist and proximal pole.[3] The volar approach also has the added risk of screw cutout through the concave volar surface of the scaphoid or through the dorsoulnar aspect of the proximal pole. The challenges of the volar approach were highlighted by a study by Levitz and Ring,[12] which attempted to quantify optimal scaphoid screw insertion for scaphoid waist fractures via a volar retrograde insertion technique with a Synthes cannulated-headed screw (Synthes, Paoli, PA). They evaluated 15 unfractured scaphoids using quantitative computer analysis of CT images. They defined the optimal screw placement as a 2 mm safe margin between the central axis of the screw and at least 5 mm of screw tip crossing the fracture site and engaging the proximal pole. They found that in all insertion planes there was a substantial concavity of the volar surface of the scaphoid, which posed a substantial potential for screw cut out. A more radial insertion point minimized this risk but this left little margin for error because the average clearance of the trapezium measured 4 mm, which is the same diameter as most scaphoid screws. They also found that the most likely place for a volarly inserted screw to perforate the articular surface is the dorsal radial surface of the scaphoid, which is exacerbated by any angular or humpback deformity. This study highlights the need to carefully fluoroscopically evaluate the dorsal radial surface of the scaphoid by gradual pronation with the wrist in slight extension. Also it shows that a relatively radial starting point facilitates placement of the screw tip in the center of the proximal pole and helps avoid the trapezium, but drilling or partial excision of the trapezium often may be necessary for optimal screw placement.

Arthroscopy can be used to help assess the vascularity of the proximal pole. To evaluate the blood supply of the proximal pole, deflate the tourniquet and place the scope in the STT portal and debride the nonunion site after infiltrating the portal sites with 2% lidocaine and 1:200,000 adrenaline. Punctate bleeding from the proximal pole will be evident (**Fig. 5**).

Arthroscopic bone grafting

Ho recently described a technique of arthroscopic-assisted bone grafting of scaphoid

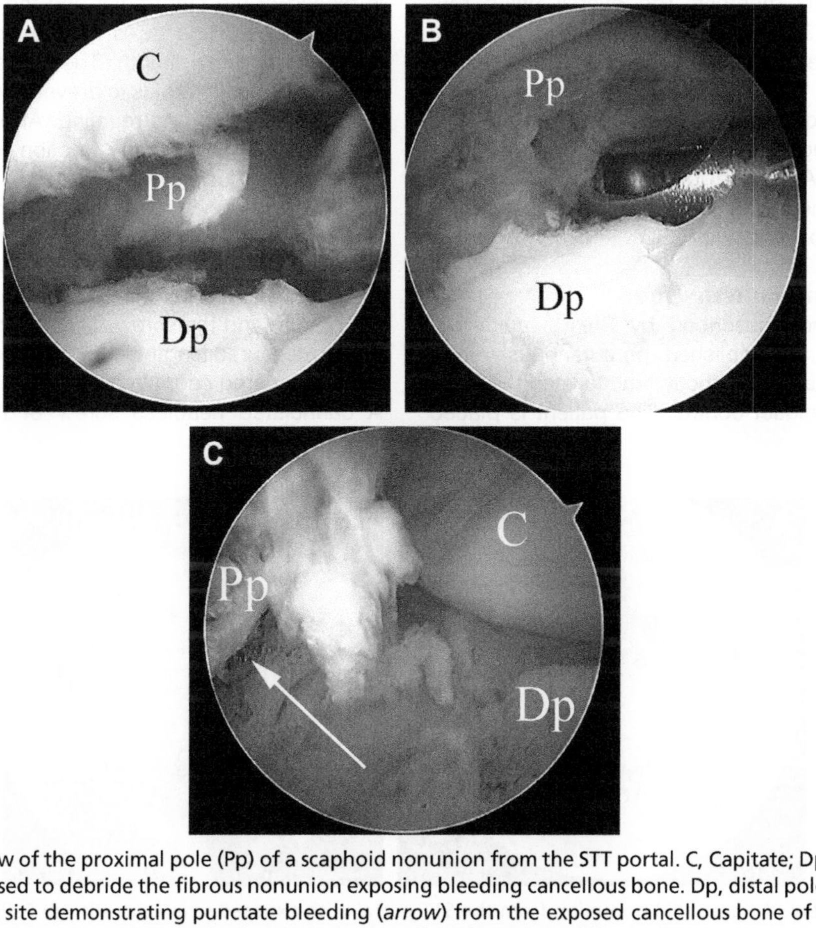

Fig. 5. (*A*) View of the proximal pole (Pp) of a scaphoid nonunion from the STT portal. C, Capitate; Dp, distal pole. (*B*) Shaver is used to debride the fibrous nonunion exposing bleeding cancellous bone. Dp, distal pole. (*C*) View of the nonunion site demonstrating punctate bleeding (*arrow*) from the exposed cancellous bone of the proximal pole (Pp). C, Capitate; Dp, distal pole. (© 2013. Slutsky. All Rights Reserved.)

nonunions.[13] The arthroscope is inserted in the MCU portal, whereas the MCR portal is used for instrumentation. The proximal nonunion site is best seen from the STT-U portal, which is radial to the extensor carpi radialis brevis tendon and ulnar to the extensor pollicus longus tendon, slightly distal to MCR portal. Loose implants (if present) are exchanged with a larger screw or multiple k-wires. Care is taken to preserve any intact cartilage or pseudocapsule over the nonunion site to avoid subsequent graft protrusion into the radiocarpal joint. Cancellous bone graft is tightly impacted into the nonunion site through an arthroscopic cannula (**Fig. 6**). His series included 37 patients with established symptomatic nonunions and 6 delayed unions with an average age of 28.7 years (range, 14–53 years). The median duration of symptoms was 8 months (range: 1–192 months). There were 5 distal third, 24 mid-third, and 14 proximal third fractures with 5 cases of previous failed surgery and 10 cases with MRI evidence of avascular necrosis. Cannulated screws were used in 20 cases and multiple K wires in 23 cases. The average follow-up was 38.3 months (range, 5–103 months). The overall union rate was 90.7% (39/43). The average time to radiological union was 12.2 weeks (6–24 weeks). Poor intraoperative bleeding of the proximal scaphoid still permitted union in 7 out of 10 cases, whereas brisk bleeding was associated with union in 29 out of 30 cases. At the final follow-up, 27 patients were pain free, whereas the average pain VAS in the remaining 16 patients was 2.53.

Volar nontraction technique

In the method described by Shin,[14] guidewire insertion is accomplished percutaneously in a freehand manner without traction and initially without tourniquet control. The patient is placed under general or regional anesthesia and then positioned supine on the operating table with the arm extended in supination on a hand table or arm board. A fluoroscopy unit is positioned over the arm board, vertical to the floor. The wrist is hyperextended over a folded towel. Two straight lines can be drawn on the skin along the longitudinal axis of the scaphoid in the anteroposterior view and the lateral view to aid in guidewire alignment. A 1-mm guidewire is introduced volarly, entering the distal scaphoid tuberosity, using a power drill, and directed along the marked lines proximally, dorsally, and ulnar-wards. The position is checked fluoroscopically to confirm that the guidewire is placed along the scaphoid axis, through the fracture site, and that it had purchased sufficient subchondral bone of the proximal pole. Although the guidewire is placed eccentrically through the distal pole, it can still pass through the central axis at the waist. A transtrapezial k-wire insertion would be required to pass through the central axis of the distal fragment, but this is not necessary. A second guidewire is inserted parallel to the first wire for rotational control. The tip of a second guidewire is placed at the entry point and the difference in length between the wires is measured to obtain the desired screw length. The guidewire can be advanced into the radius to prevent it from backing out during drilling and reaming. At this point, the hand is suspended in the traction tower and an arthroscopic survey is performed. The reduction can be fine tuned under arthroscopic control. Once the fracture is satisfactorily reduced, the arm is taken out of traction. A 2- to 3-mm incision is made at the base of the guidewire for passage of the reamer and the screw. The scaphoid is drilled to the measured length under fluoroscopic control using a tapered cannulated drill and then tapped. A cannulated headless screw of the surgeons

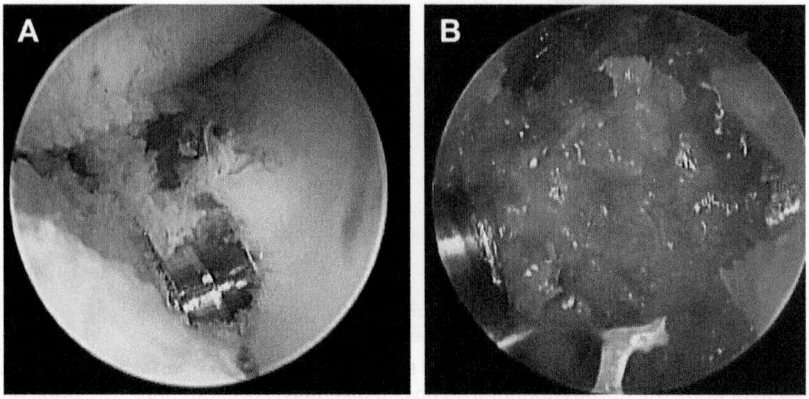

Fig. 6. (*A*) View of a scaphoid nonunion from the STT portal with exposed screw threads. (*B*) Following arthroscopic bone grafting. (© 2013. Slutsky. All Rights Reserved.)

preference is then hand inserted under fluoroscopic guidance. Similar to the dorsal approach, the screw should be no closer than 2 mm from the proximal pole articular surface and well buried in the distal pole.

Volar traction technique

Haddad and Goddard described a volar percutaneous scaphoid fixation method using a cannulated screw.[15] The patient is placed supine on an operating table with the arm in traction. The hand is suspended by the thumb alone in a single Chinese finger trap with no countertraction. This position extends the scaphoid, and ulnar deviates the wrist to improve access to the distal pole of the scaphoid. Importantly, it permits free rotation of the hand throughout the operation and the scaphoid remains in the center of the X-ray field throughout. He infiltrates the proposed entry point of the guidewire with 2 cc of 2% lidocaine and 1:200,000 adrenaline. The use of a tourniquet is optional. The image intensifier C arm is turned to a horizontal position and positioned so that the wrist is in the central axis. With the image intensifier in this position, it is possible to screen the scaphoid continuously around the axis of the radial column. K-wires can be inserted and used as joysticks to manipulate the fragments into position as necessary. The quality of the reduction can then be checked radiographically and if necessary arthroscopically without disturbing the overall setup. The guidewire entry point is located using a 12-gauge IV needle introduced on the volar radial aspect of the wrist just radial to and distal to the scaphoid tuberosity, and the needle is used to lever the distal pole of the scaphoid more radial to facilitate screw insertion (**Fig. 7**). The forearm is rotated under fluoroscopy to line up the needle along the long axis of the scaphoid in all planes so that the guidewire exits the proximal pole just radial to the scapholunate junction. The entry point can be changed by up to 1 mm by rotating the IV cannula. The guidewire is then inserted through the needle and drilled across the fracture site

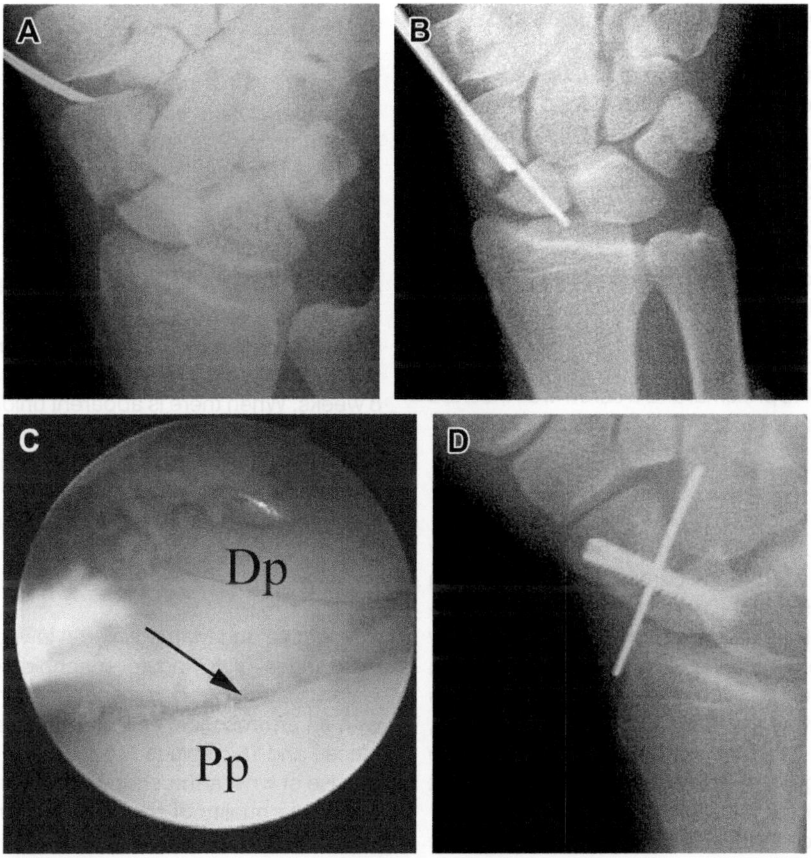

Fig. 7. (*A*) Positioning of an 18-gauge needle in the distal scaphoid pole under fluoroscopy. (*B*) Insertion of a guidewire. Second guidewire is used to manipulate and reduce the proximal fragment. (*C*) View of the reduction of the scaphoid fracture (*arrow*) through the MCR portal. Dp, distal pole; Pp, proximal pole. (*D*) Completed construct. (© 2013. Slutsky. All Rights Reserved.)

under fluoroscopy, stopping just short of the proximal pole. A small incision is made over the guidewire, followed by screw insertion. The length of the screw is determined using a second guidewire of the same length up the distal cortex of the scaphoid and undersized by 4 mm. The guidewire is then advanced through the proximal pole to exit on the dorsal aspect of the wrist to minimize the risk of inadvertent withdrawal. The arthroscopic survey is performed along with any fine tuning of the reduction, followed by reaming and screw insertion.

Hybrid technique

Pirela-Cruz and coauthors[16] described a hybrid technique for a Herbert B-2 fracture with a standard-sized cannulated Acutrak screw; this combines the ease of dorsal guidewire placement with the advantages of volar screw insertion. Using Slade's technique[17] the forearm is pronated and the wrist is radially deviated and flexed over a bump of towels until the proximal and distal poles are superimposed on fluoroscopy to create a cortical ring sign. A double-ended guidewire is drilled into the center of the proximal pole of the scaphoid. With correct placement, the guidewire should appear as a dot within the center of a circle. Once the correct position of the guidewire is obtained, the wire is advanced out through the volar side at the tuberosity of the scaphoid until the guidewire is located within the proximal pole. The authors were usually able to obtain a satisfactory dorsal-central position without drilling through the trapezium. The wrist was then placed into extension and ulnar deviation and the guidewire is advanced into the radius to prevent dislodgement after the length of the screw is determined. The scaphoid was reamed to within 2 to 3 mm of the proximal and a screw was inserted under fluoroscopic control.

COMPLICATIONS

Screw cut out, tendon injury, or overly long screw lengths are common complications following percutaneous dorsal screw implantation. Adamany and colleagues[18] performed a cadaver study of dorsal percutaneous screw insertion, seating the screw under fluoroscopy. The structures most at risk were the posterior interosseous nerve, which was 2.2 mm from the guidewire, the extensor digitorum communis to the index at 2.2 mm, and the extensor indicis proprius at 3.1 mm. They incorrectly placed the screw above the subchondral bone despite live fluoroscopy in 2 specimens. The use of arthroscopy however can protect against screw prominence. Weinberg and colleagues[19] performed a study on percutaneous dorsal guidewire insertion in 40 cadaver arms. No nerve or vessel injuries were observed but tendons however were injured in 5 specimens including the extensor pollicis longus tendon (2), the extensor carpi radialis tendon (2) and the extensor digitorum tendon (1). They noted that these soft tissue injuries could be avoided using a mini-open dorsal approach.

Bushnell and colleagues[20] reviewed a single surgeon's complications following dorsal percutaneous screw insertion of 24 patients with nondisplaced scaphoid waist fractures. They reported 1 nonunion, 3 cases involving hardware problems, 1 case of a postoperative fracture of the proximal pole of the scaphoid, and 2 cases of intraoperative equipment breakage. Slade, however, reported only 2 complications in 234 cases: 1 case of delayed healing and 1 case of recurrent dislocation of a volar transscaphoid perilunate dislocation.[2] These 2 studies emphasizes that there is a significant learning curve with percutaneous techniques and that many of the complications are operator dependent.

POST-OPERATIVE CARE

The tourniquet is then deflated and the skin incisions are closed with subcuticular sutures and Steri-Strips. The incisions are infiltrated with 0.25% Marcaine and the joint can be injected with 5 mg of Duramorph for patient comfort but an axillary block is preferred. A short arm thumb spica splint is applied after wound closure. The post-operative dressing is changed at 1 week. Although some investigators allow immediate and unrestricted motion, the author prefers to immobilize the wrist in a short arm thumb spica cast for 6 to 8 weeks. When there is apparent union on the plain radiographic views, a longitudinal CT scan is performed to confirm that there is bridging callus on at least 3 cuts. Wrist motion and progressive strengthening exercises are then instituted.

OUTCOMES

Martinache and Mathoulin[21] reviewed their results of a series of 37 acute scaphoid fractures that were treated by percutaneous screw insertion with an arthroscopic assist. There were 22 undisplaced and 15 displaced fractures. In all the cases, the use of wrist arthroscopy allowed the authors to check the quality of the reduction and the screw position. Bony union was achieved in all of the cases, within a median time of 62 days (range 45–80). The functional recovery of the operated wrists was reported to be good with an average return to work 21 days after the surgery.

Slade recently reported a consecutive series of 234 fractures treated with percutaneous screw fixation using a dorsal approach.[2] The cases included 108 scaphoid nonunions (10 with a humpback deformity) and 126 acute injuries comprised of 65 proximal pole fractures, 67 grossly displaced fractures, 12 transscaphoid perilunate dislocations, 4 transscaphoid transcapitate fractures, and 10 combined scaphoid and distal radius fractures. In each case arthroscopy was used to verify the quality of the reduction. CT scans confirmed that 125/126 acute

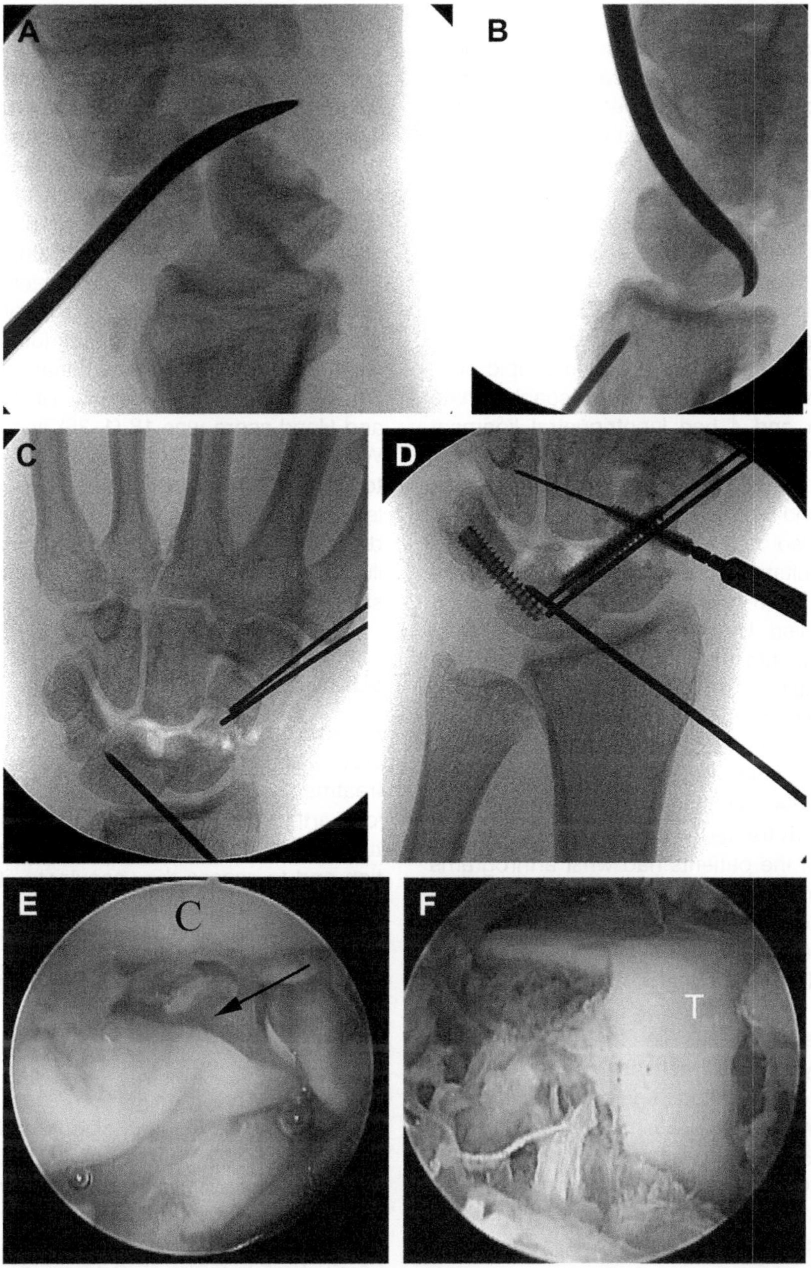

Fig. 8. Arthroscopic assisted transscaphoid perilunate dislocation. (*A*) Lateral view showing percutaneous insertion of elevator over dorsal lip of dislocated lunate. (*B*) Elevator is used to lever the lunate into a reduced position. (*C*) Percutaneous insertion of scaphoid guidewires. Note radiolunate k-wire. (*D*) Percutaneous insertion of scaphoid screw as well as temporary screw fixation of scaphocapitate and lunotriquetral joints. (*E*) Tear of the space of Poirier (*arrow*) seen from the MCR portal. C, capitate. (*F*) Osteochondral fracture of triquetrum (T) seen through the MCU portal. (© 2013. Slutsky. All Rights Reserved.)

fractures and 98/108 nonunions healed. The study demonstrated the utility of arthroscopy, which aided the fracture reduction in 67 displaced fractures in addition to the 10 humpback deformities. Slade also used arthroscopy to assess the vascularity of the proximal pole by inserting the scope in the screw tract of the proximal fragment after reaming and then releasing the tourniquet to gauge the amount of bleeding.

Arthroscopy is helpful for assessing concomitant soft tissue injuries with scaphoid fractures. Caloia and colleagues[1] performed an arthroscopic examination on 24 patients with acute scaphoid fractures who were treated with percutaneous screw fixation through a dorsal approach. The mean age was 32 years (range, 17–75 years). Fifteen of the 24 patients had an associated ligamentous or chondral injury. In a similar study, Shih and colleagues[22] reviewed 15 patients with an acute scaphoid fracture treated by percutaneous screw fixation under an arthroscopic control. Two patients had a partial scapholunate ligament tear and 4 had lunotriquetral ligament tear, which were debrided and k-wired. Five patients had a triangular fibrocartilage complex (TFCC) tear and 6 patients had chondral fractures. There were also 5 patients with injuries to the radioscaphocapitate ligament or long radiolunate ligament. At the 28-month follow-up all of the fractures had healed. Using the Modified Mayo Wrist score, 11 patients had excellent results and 4 had good results.

Associated soft tissue injuries represent a higher severity of trauma and negatively affect outcomes following scaphoid fracture. Wong and colleagues[23] studied 52 patients with scaphoid fractures who were treated with percutaneous screw fixation. All of the patients had wrist arthrograms and 22 underwent arthroscopy. Eighteen patients were found to have additional soft tissue injures, which included 4 scapholunate ligament tears, 8 lunotriquetral ligament tears, 2 combined tears, and 3 TFCC tears. There was a noticeable difference in the outcomes in that the median-modified Mayo wrist score was 95 in the patients without any associated ligament injuries as compared with a score of 85 in patients with associated ligament injuries. Arthroscopy assist allows the surgeon to recognize, potentially treat these injuries, and provides a better understanding of the expected post-operative course.

TRANSSCAPHOID PERILUNATE DISLOCATION

There has been some recent work into the use of arthroscopy and transscaphoid perilunate fracture dislocations (**Fig. 8**). Wong and Ip[24] reviewed the results in 21 patients with a mean age of 29 years who underwent a closed reduction of the carpus, percutaneous screw fixation of the scaphoid fracture, and multiple k-wire fixation of the carpal dissociation. There was a 95% union rate with a mean time of 16 weeks. The radiographic alignment of the carpus was satisfactory in 17 out of 21 cases. The average Mayo wrist score was 80 with 3 excellent and 2 poor results. They had 1 patient with asymptomatic dorsal intercalated segment instability deformity, 2 with radiographic evidence of midcarpal arthritis, and 1 scaphoid nonunion, which required revision surgery and bone grafting. Jeon and colleagues[25] treated 20 patients who had an acute dorsal perilunate dislocation (5) or fracture dislocation (15) with an arthroscopic scaphoid screw insertion, followed by k-wiring of the carpus for 10 weeks. At a mean follow-up of 31.2 months, the mean flexion was 51° (25–70), mean extension 53° (30–70), radial deviation 17° (10–26), and ulnar deviation 30° (18–42). The mean Disability of Arm, Shoulder and Hand score was 18 (1–36) and Patient-rated Wrist Evaluation score was 30 (5–52). According to modified Mayo wrist scores, there were 3 excellent, 8 good, 87 fair, and 2 poor results. Nonunion developed in 2 patients with a transscaphoid perilunate injury; 1 of the 2 underwent scaphoid excision and midcarpal fusion.

SUMMARY

Arthroscopy allows the surgeon to use smaller incisions and still have predictable outcomes in the treatment of scaphoid fractures. Similar to large joint arthroscopy, the ability to visualize the fracture site allows one to not only fine tune the reduction and to assess the vascularity of the fracture fragments but to evaluate and treat any associated soft tissue injuries that may affect the end result. Specialized equipment and a basic knowledge of wrist arthroscopy however are required.

REFERENCES

1. Caloia MF, Gallino RN, Caloia H, et al. Incidence of ligamentous and other injuries associated with scaphoid fractures during arthroscopically assisted reduction and percutaneous fixation. Arthroscopy 2008;24:754–9.
2. Slade JF 3rd, Gillon T. Retrospective review of 234 scaphoid fractures and nonunions treated with arthroscopy for union and complications. Scand J Surg 2008;97:280–9.
3. Chan KW, McAdams TR. Central screw placement in percutaneous screw scaphoid fixation: a cadaveric

comparison of proximal and distal techniques. J Hand Surg Am 2004;29:74–9.
4. Jeon IH, Kochhar H, Lee BW, et al. Percutaneous screw fixation for scaphoid nonunion in skeletally immature patients: a report of two cases. J Hand Surg Am 2008;33:656–9.
5. McCallister WV, Knight J, Kaliappan R, et al. Central placement of the screw in simulated fractures of the scaphoid waist: a biomechanical study. J Bone Joint Surg Am 2003;85:72–7.
6. Dodds SD, Panjabi MM, Slade JF 3rd. Screw fixation of scaphoid fractures: a biomechanical assessment of screw length and screw augmentation. J Hand Surg Am 2006;31:405–13.
7. Trumble TE, Clarke T, Kreder HJ. Non-union of the scaphoid. Treatment with cannulated screws compared with treatment with Herbert screws. J Bone Joint Surg Am 1996;78:1829–37.
8. Menapace KA, Larabee L, Arnoczky SP, et al. Anatomic placement of the Herbert-Whipple screw in scaphoid fractures: a cadaver study. J Hand Surg Am 2001;26:883–92.
9. Leventhal EL, Wolfe SW, Walsh EF, et al. A computational approach to the "optimal" screw axis location and orientation in the scaphoid bone. J Hand Surg Am 2009;34:677–84.
10. Heinzelmann AD, Archer G, Bindra RR. Anthropometry of the human scaphoid. J Hand Surg Am 2007; 32:1005–8.
11. Slade JF 3rd, Dodds SD. Minimally invasive management of scaphoid nonunions. Clin Orthop Relat Res 2006;445:108–19.
12. Levitz S, Ring D. Retrograde (volar) scaphoid screw insertion-a quantitative computed tomographic analysis. J Hand Surg Am 2005;30:543–8.
13. Ho P. Arthroscopic bone grafting in scaphoid non union & delayed union. In: Slutsky DJ, Slade JF, editors. The scaphoid. New York: Thieme; 2010. p. 131–43.
14. Shin AY, Hofmeister EP. Percutaneous fixation of stable scaphoid fractures. Tech Hand Up Extrem Surg 2004;8:87–94.
15. Haddad FS, Goddard NJ. Acute percutaneous scaphoid fixation. A pilot study. J Bone Joint Surg Br 1998;80:95–9.
16. Pirela-Cruz MA, Battista V, Burnette S, et al. A technical note on percutaneous scaphoid fixation using a hybrid technique. J Orthop Trauma 2005;19: 570–3.
17. Slade JF 3rd, Jaskwhich D. Percutaneous fixation of scaphoid fractures. Hand Clin 2001;17:553–74.
18. Adamany DC, Mikola EA, Fraser BJ. Percutaneous fixation of the scaphoid through a dorsal approach: an anatomic study. J Hand Surg Am 2008;33:327–31.
19. Weinberg AM, Pichler W, Grechenig S, et al. The percutaneous antegrade scaphoid fracture fixation–a safe method? Injury 2009;40:642–4.
20. Bushnell BD, McWilliams AD, Messer TM. Complications in dorsal percutaneous cannulated screw fixation of nondisplaced scaphoid waist fractures. J Hand Surg Am 2007;32:827–33.
21. Martinache X, Mathoulin C. Percutaneous fixation of scaphoid fractures with arthroscopic assistance. Chir Main 2006;25(Suppl 1):S171–7 [in French].
22. Shih JT, Lee HM, Hou YT, et al. Results of arthroscopic reduction and percutaneous fixation for acute displaced scaphoid fractures. Arthroscopy 2005;21:620–6.
23. Wong TC, Yip TH, Wu WC. Carpal ligament injuries with acute scaphoid fractures - a combined wrist injury. J Hand Surg Br 2005;30:415–8.
24. Wong TC, Ip FK. Minimally invasive management of trans-scaphoid perilunate fracture-dislocations. Hand Surg 2008;13:159–65.
25. Jeon IH, Kim HJ, Min WK, et al. Arthroscopically assisted percutaneous fixation for trans-scaphoid perilunate fracture dislocation. J Hand Surg Eur Vol 2010;35:664–8.

Index

Note: Page numbers of article titles are in **boldface** type.

Hand Clin 30 (2014) 105–107
http://dx.doi.org/10.1016/S0749-0712(13)00103-0
0749-0712/14/$ – see front matter

Printed and bound by CPI Group (UK) Ltd, Croydon, CR0 4YY
03/10/2024
01040309-0008